KENZ ~~RUNS~~ THE WORLD

BRIAN CLEVEN

With Motivational Messages From:

Gwen Jorgensen

Chris Nikic

Sika Henry

Dave McGillivray

ILLUSTRATED BY EDD

DEDICATION

To Amy, Natasha, and Kenzie,

The love and joy that you bring to my life drives me to make you proud in everything I do. You are truly my greatest blessings from above!

Be Kind, Be Brave,

And Always Believe,

Anything Is Possible!

To my parents Russ and Kathy,

I could never **THANK YOU** enough for everything you have done for me. Your love and support have literally opened the entire world to me, and you have guided me to success.

To friends and family,

Thank you for the joy you have brought to my life. You are loved and appreciated.

To everyone,

Never forget to enjoy the journey!

Copyright © 2024 by Brian Cleven

All rights reserved, including the right to reproduce, distribute, or transmit in any form or by any means.

ISBN: 979-8-9895546-3-8

MOTIVATIONAL MESSAGES FROM FAMOUS FRIENDS

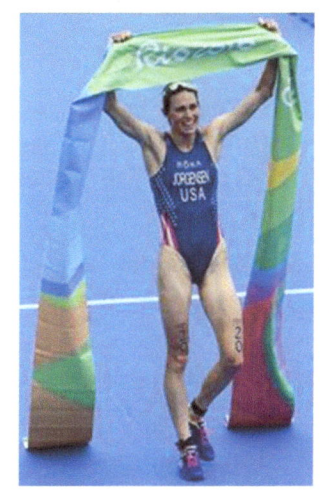

"Running has taken me from a small town in Wisconsin all the way to the top of the Olympic Podium in Rio De Janeiro as a Gold Medal Winner in Triathlon. Along the way I have made fabulous friends, traveled the world, and have found great courage within myself on the journey. Dreams start by seeing and then believing followed by taking action to reach them. Just like in this book with Kenzie and her friends, runners can come in all shapes, sizes, abilities, and live anywhere. As a mom I love it when my children find a book that captures their attention and helps them learn and dream. Great potential and ability lie within us all so dream big, work hard, and leave a positive impact on the world around you. Please enjoy this trip around the world with Kenzie and all her new friends." **-Gwen Jorgensen**

Olympic Gold Medalist, World Champion Triathlete, Mom, Accountant

"At age 18 I was overweight, out of shape, and could not run 100 yards. I was isolated and alone. I started to run 100 yards to get in shape and make some friends with a goal to get 1% better every day. 3 years later, I became the first Special Olympics athlete and the first person with Down Syndrome to finish an IRONMAN triathlon. Now I have friends and I run all over the world with them. I have completed all 6 world marathon majors, the IRONMAN World Championship in Hawaii, and so many more. I am seeing and learning about the wonderful world we live in because of running. Please enjoy this journey with Kenzie and her new friends and believe that you can accomplish your dreams too if you work hard to reach them." **-Chris Nikic**

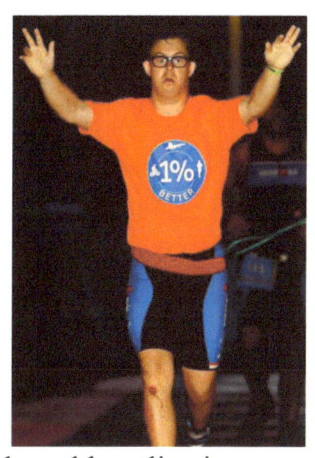

IRONMAN, Six Star Finisher, Two-time ESPY Winner, Public Speaker

"I love taking on BIG challenges and the sense of accomplishment when you reach the finish line, but I also run to make a difference. As an African American female running has helped me bring awareness and help improve inclusion both in the sport of triathlon and in the running world. One of the highlights of my life was the day that I earned my "PRO CARD" and became the first female African American Professional Triathlete which opened the door for women of color to follow in my footsteps. Running has taken me around the world from Hawaii where I finished the IRONMAN World Championship to South Africa for the Comrades Marathon and even to the Civil Rights March Path in Alabama for a 51-mile Ultra Distance run. Reaching success in anything takes time, effort, and dedication, but if you set the goal, believe, and work hard you can accomplish your dreams. I truly believe that "if you see it, you can be it" so I love all the diverse friends Kenzie meets on her exciting journey around the world!" **-Sika Henry**

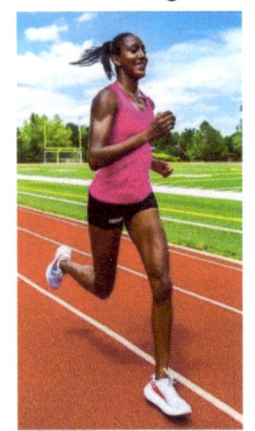

First Female African American Professional Triathlete, Ultra Distance Runner, Customer Analytics Specialist

"Running has always played a very important role in my life. In my younger years after High School, I challenged myself and ran coast to coast across the whole United States. I kept running and as of 2024, I have finished 52 Boston Marathons while being the Race Director for many of them. Never a person to turn down a challenge, I even ran 7 marathons in 7 days on all 7 continents, so I love all the amazing places Kenzie visits in this book. Running has helped me stay motivated to remain physically active, but also has opened the whole world to me. A run may last minutes or hours, but the friendships and memories you make last a lifetime. Parents and children please enjoy this fantastic journey with Kenzie and her new friends!" **-Dave McGillivray**

Boston Marathon Race Director, Endurance Legend

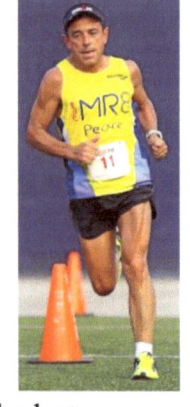

AUSTRALIA, JAPAN, USA, FRANCE

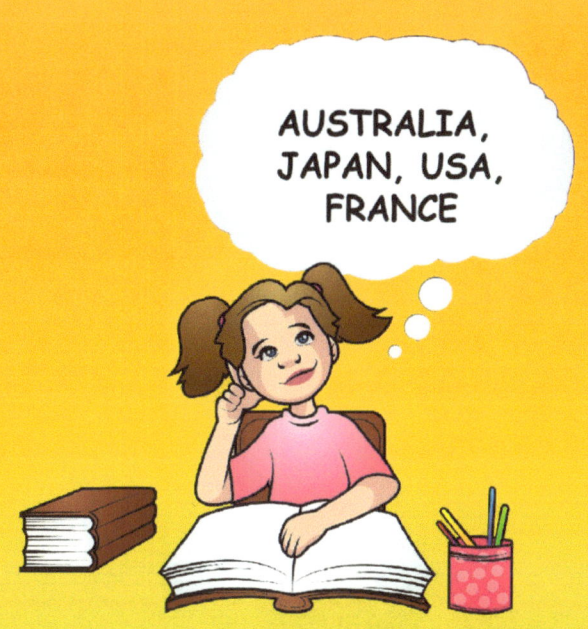

In this book Kenzie runs to feel free, to explore, and to live her life to the fullest! On her trip around the world, she meets new friends who speak different languages, wear different clothes, eat different foods, and may even follow a different religion. Friends can come in all shapes, sizes, skin colors, ages, and with different physical abilities. Learning about and celebrating our differences makes traveling and meeting new friends such an exciting opportunity!

Your life should not be judged by the clothes you wear or the car you drive, but rather by the kindness you show others and the memories you make. Be sure to check out the flag of each country in the top left corner of each page and where the country is located on the globe at the bottom right corner. If you love a page and want to learn more about the location, please scan the QR code. Children and parents, please enjoy this trip around the world with Kenzie and all her new friends.

What to look for on each page:

Flag of the country   Location on the globe   QR Code to learn more
(Top left corner)   (Bottom right corner)   (Bottom right or left)

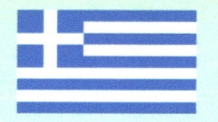

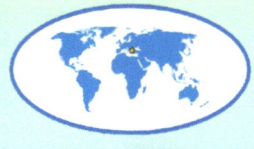

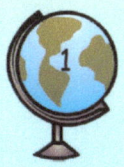

HOBBITON
NEW ZEALAND

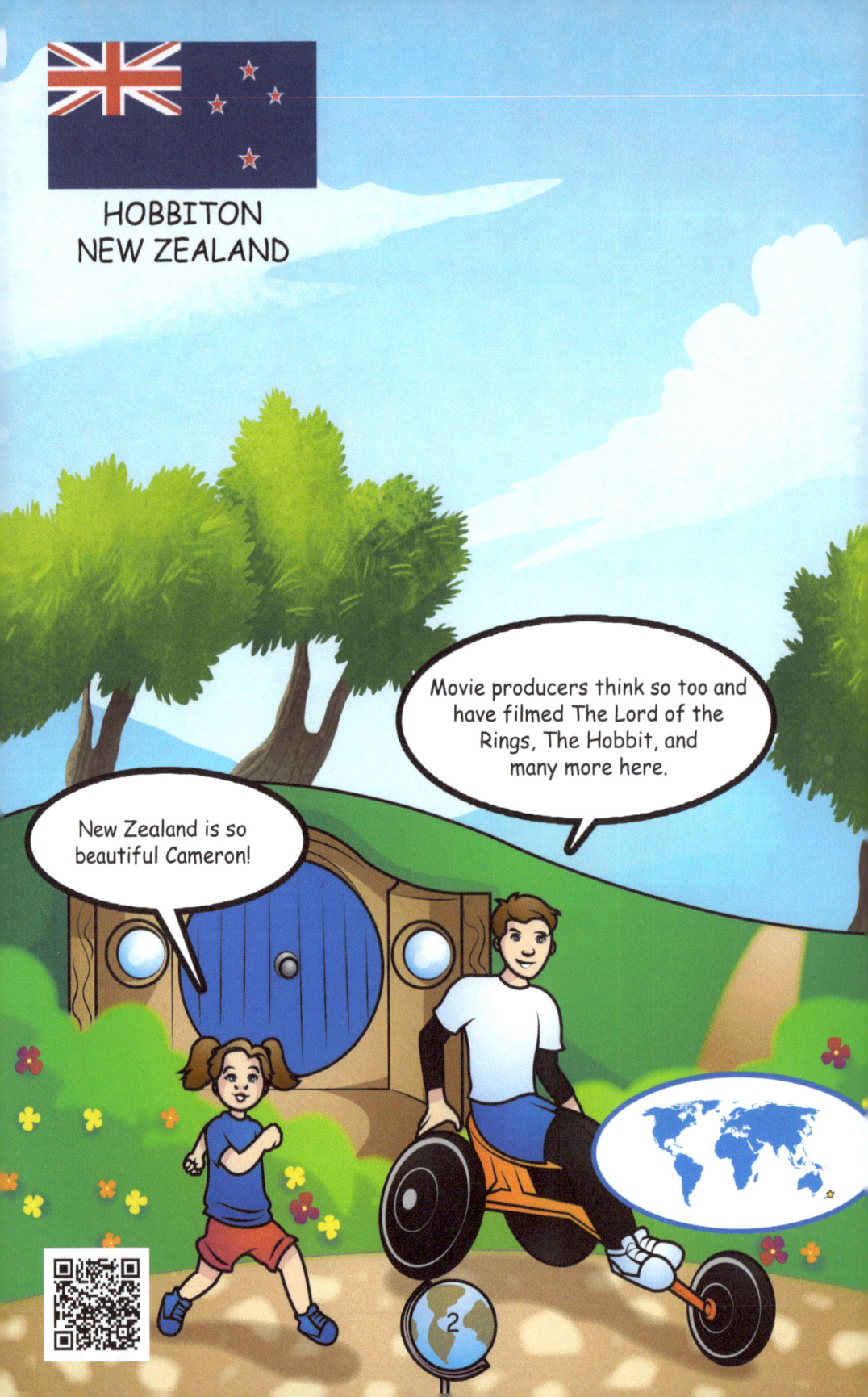

New Zealand is so beautiful Cameron!

Movie producers think so too and have filmed The Lord of the Rings, The Hobbit, and many more here.

SYDNEY
AUSTRALIA

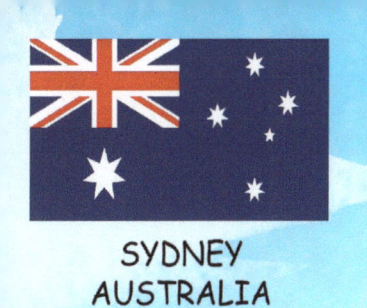

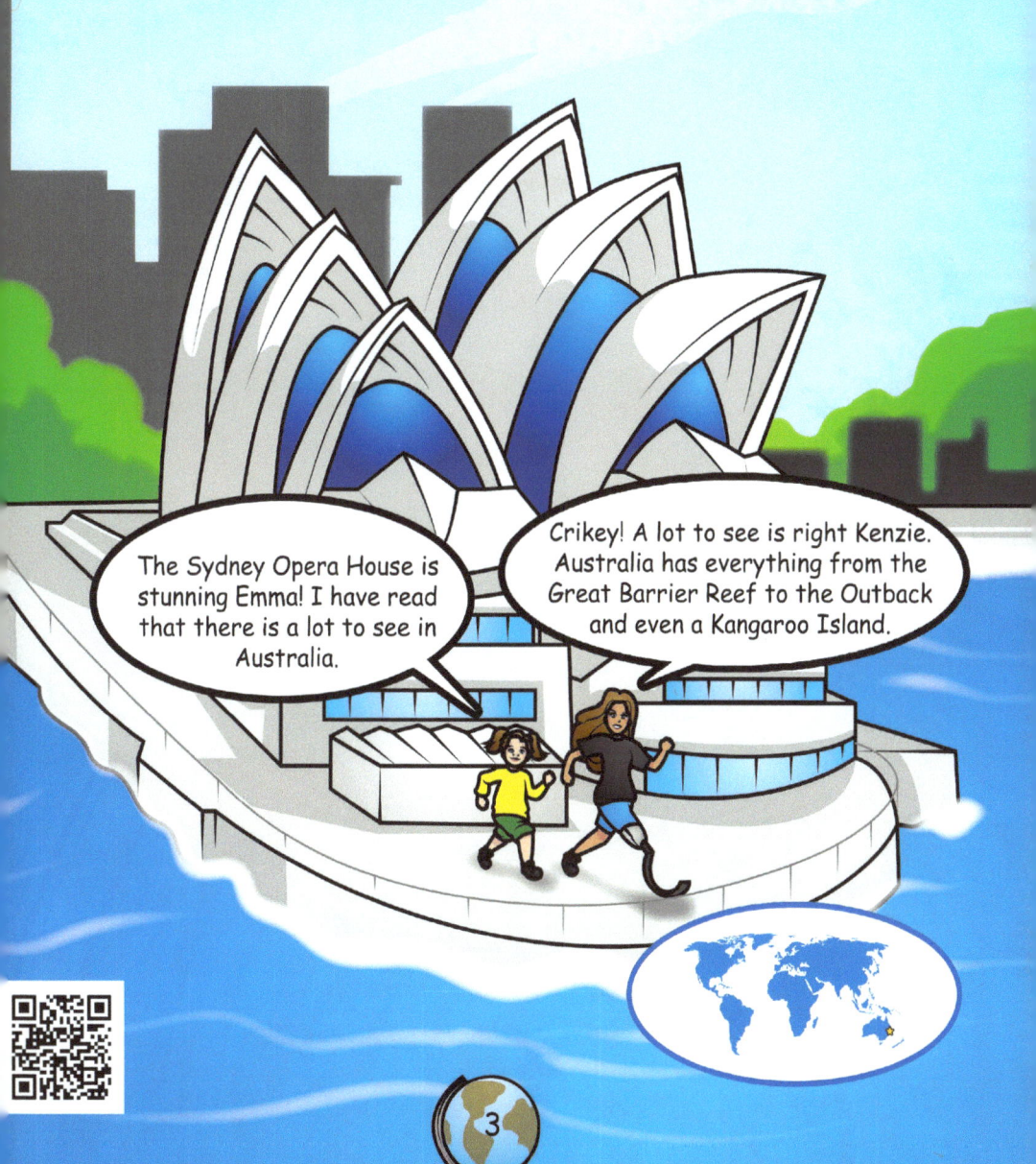

The Sydney Opera House is stunning Emma! I have read that there is a lot to see in Australia.

Crikey! A lot to see is right Kenzie. Australia has everything from the Great Barrier Reef to the Outback and even a Kangaroo Island.

3

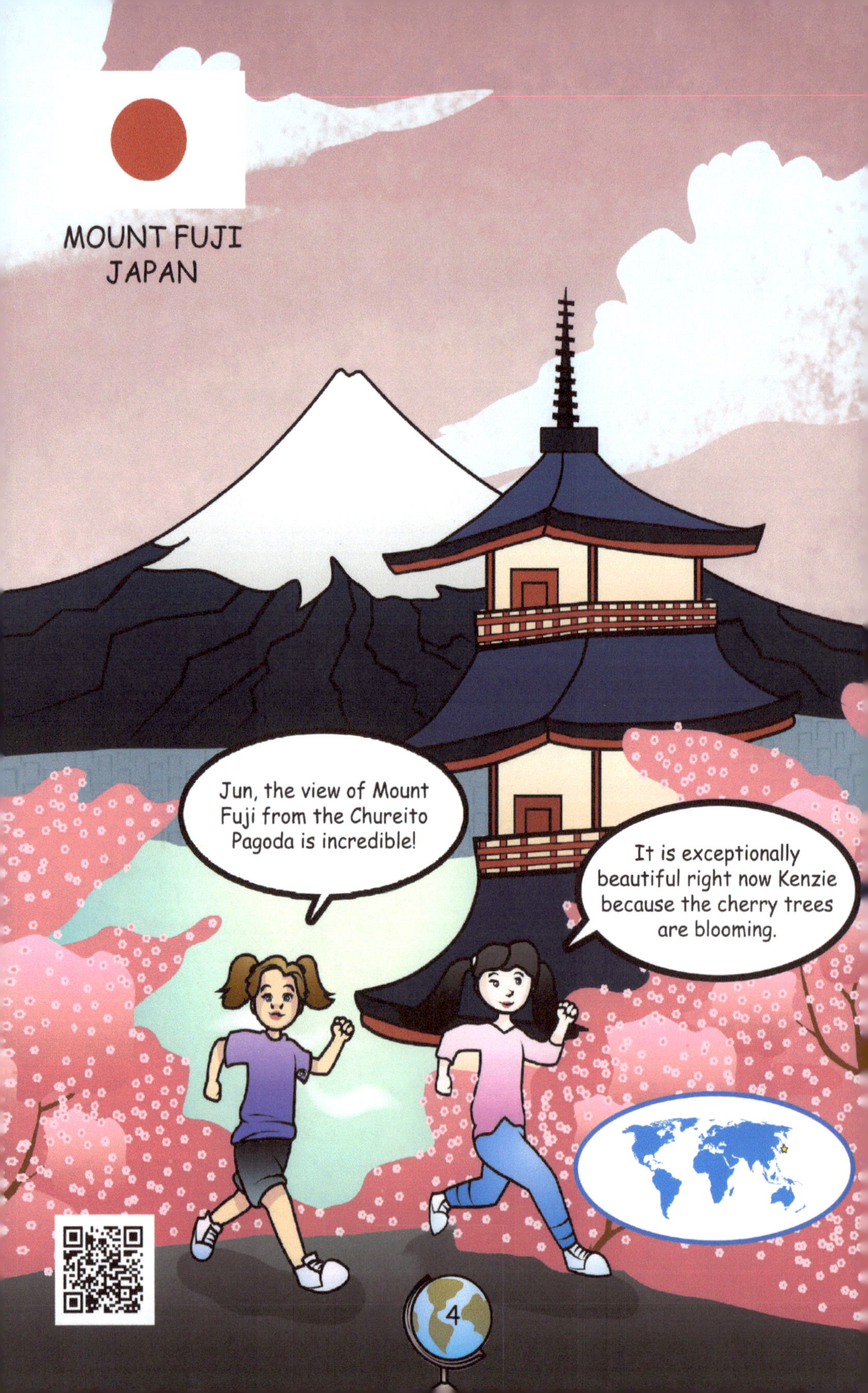
MOUNT FUJI
JAPAN
Jun, the view of Mount Fuji from the Chureito Pagoda is incredible!
It is exceptionally beautiful right now Kenzie because the cherry trees are blooming.

GREAT WALL
CHINA

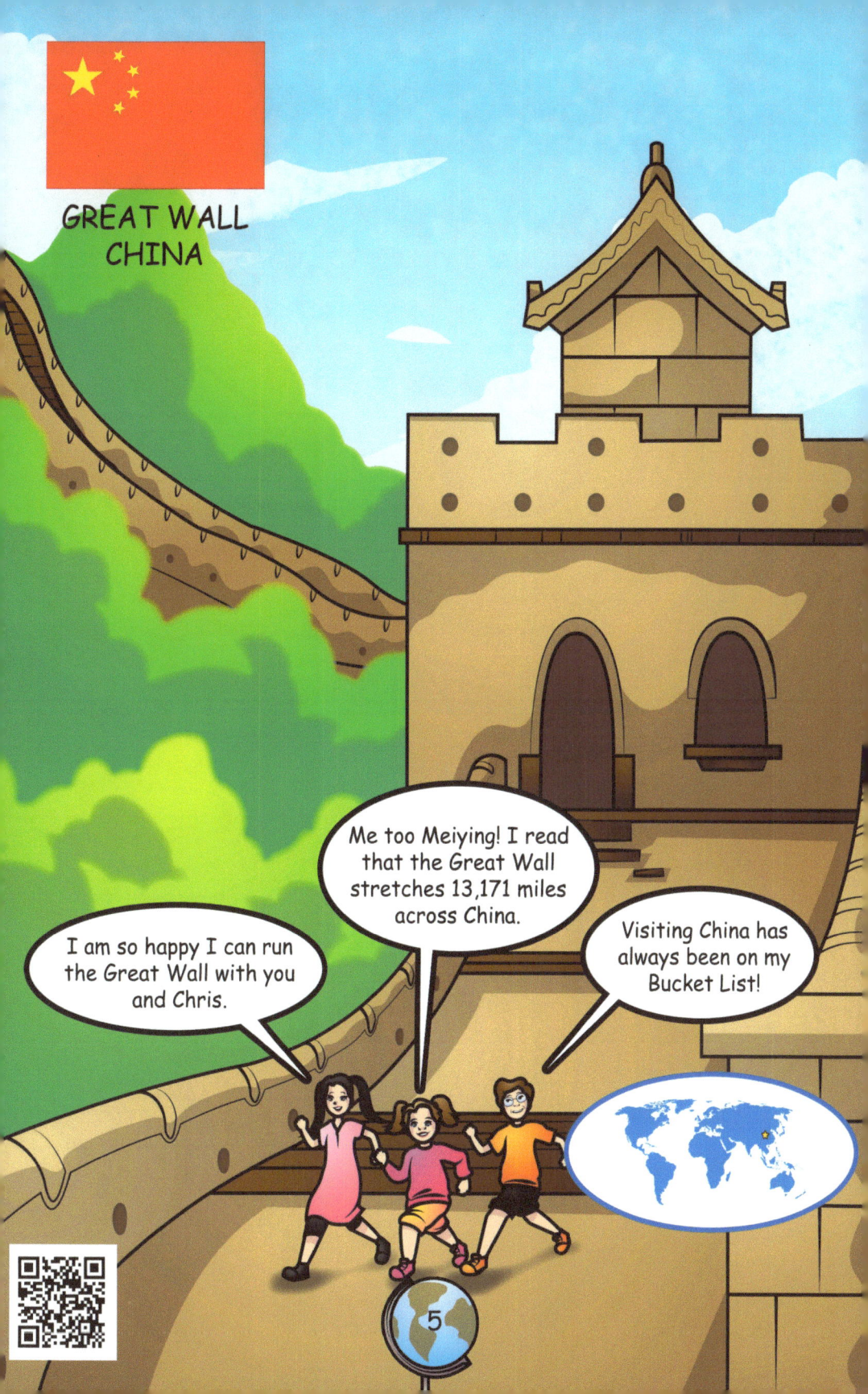

I am so happy I can run the Great Wall with you and Chris.

Me too Meiying! I read that the Great Wall stretches 13,171 miles across China.

Visiting China has always been on my Bucket List!

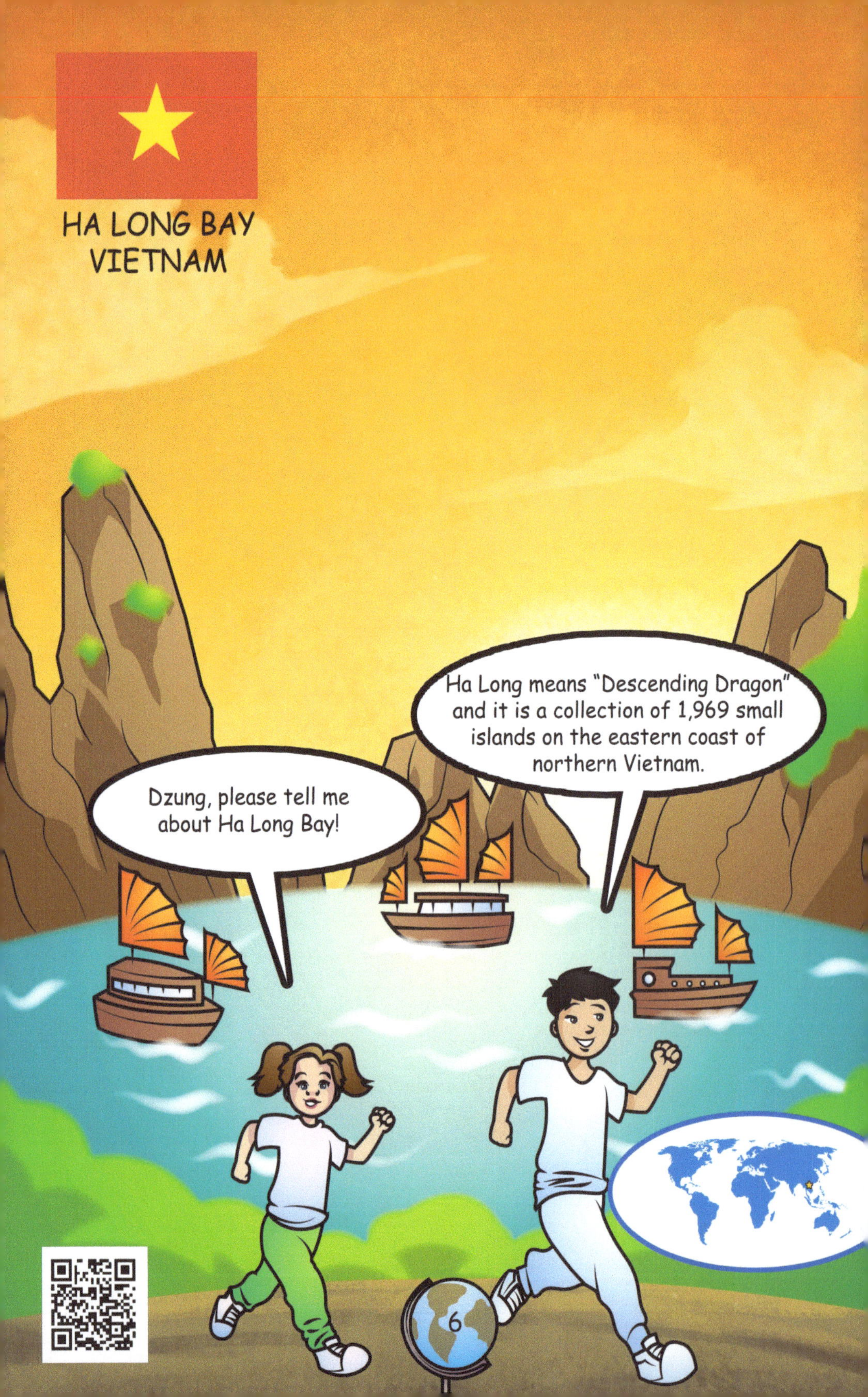
HA LONG BAY
VIETNAM
Dzung, please tell me about Ha Long Bay!
Ha Long means "Descending Dragon" and it is a collection of 1,969 small islands on the eastern coast of northern Vietnam.

ANGKOR WAT CAMBODIA

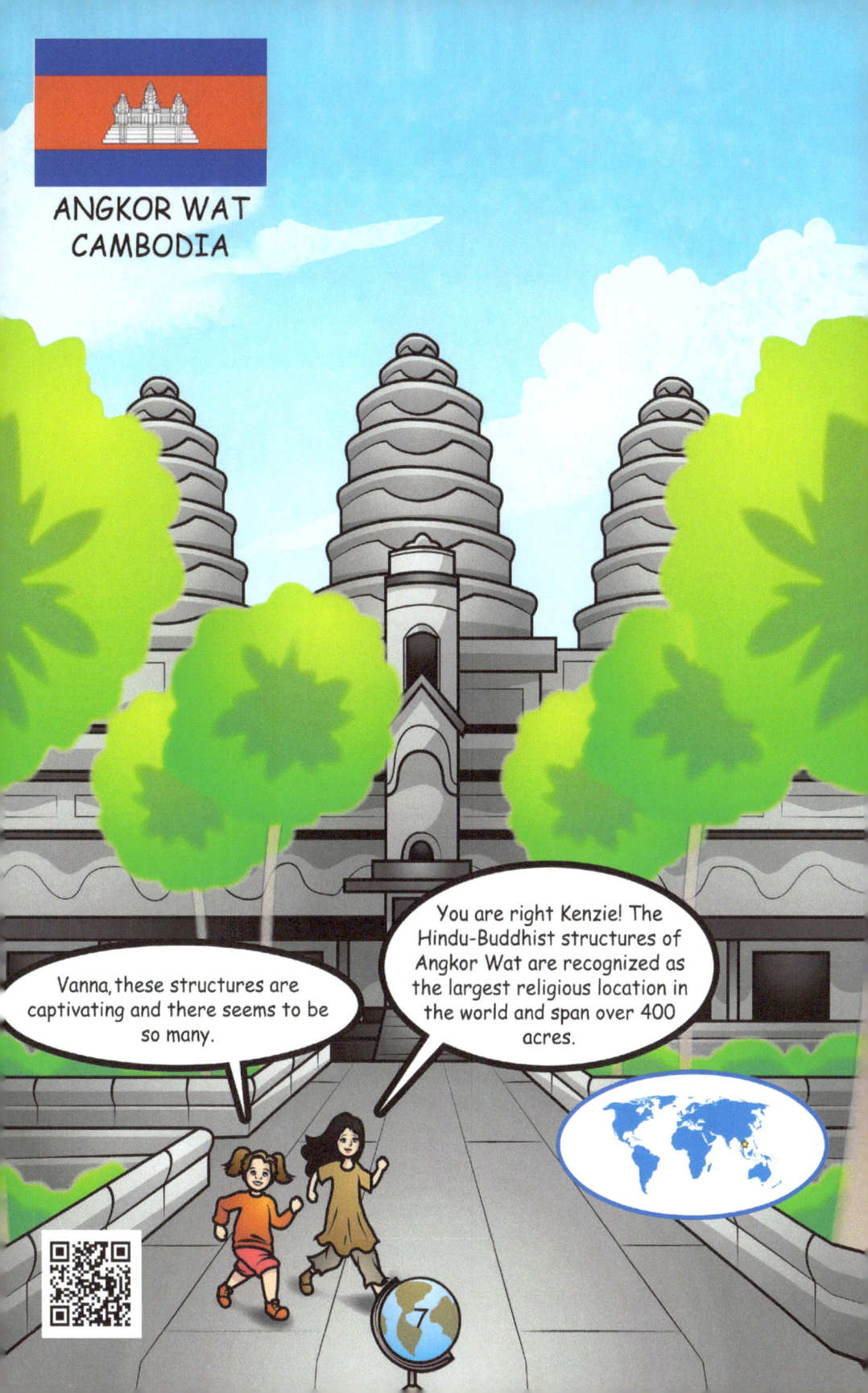

Vanna, these structures are captivating and there seems to be so many.

You are right Kenzie! The Hindu-Buddhist structures of Angkor Wat are recognized as the largest religious location in the world and span over 400 acres.

TAJ MAHAL
INDIA

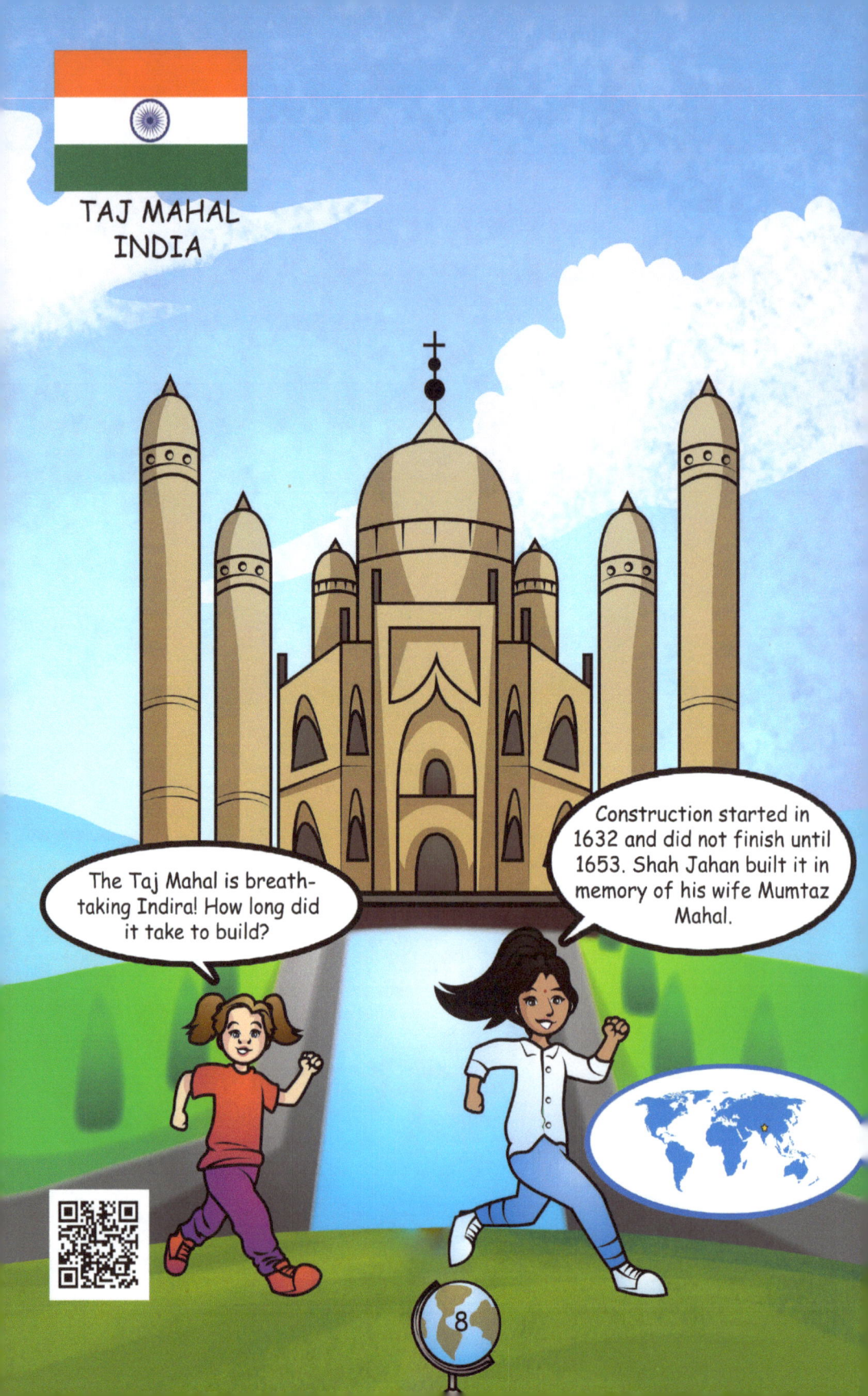

The Taj Mahal is breathtaking Indira! How long did it take to build?

Construction started in 1632 and did not finish until 1653. Shah Jahan built it in memory of his wife Mumtaz Mahal.

DAVID GAREJI MONASTERY GEORGIA

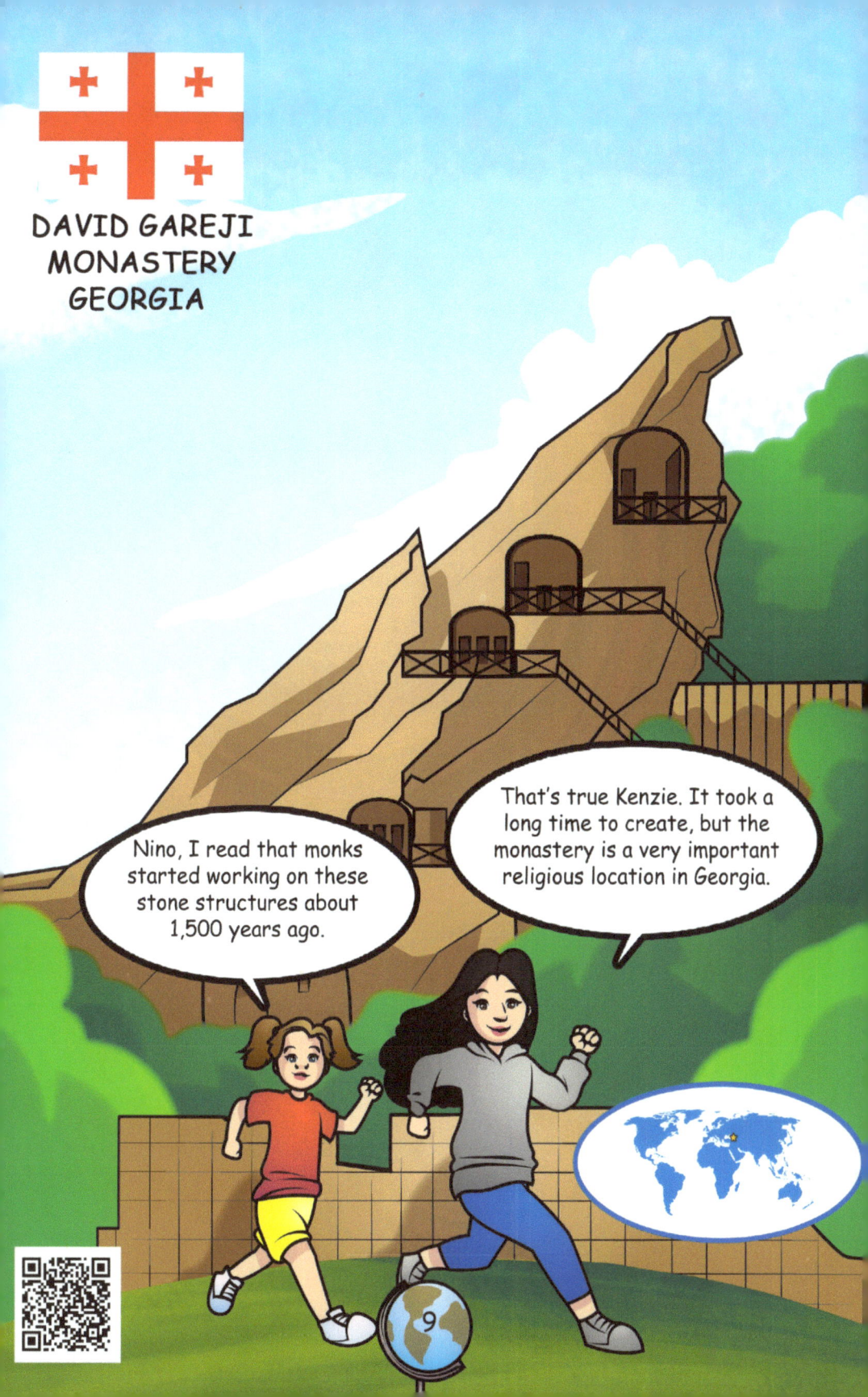

Nino, I read that monks started working on these stone structures about 1,500 years ago.

That's true Kenzie. It took a long time to create, but the monastery is a very important religious location in Georgia.

CAPPADOCIA TURKEY

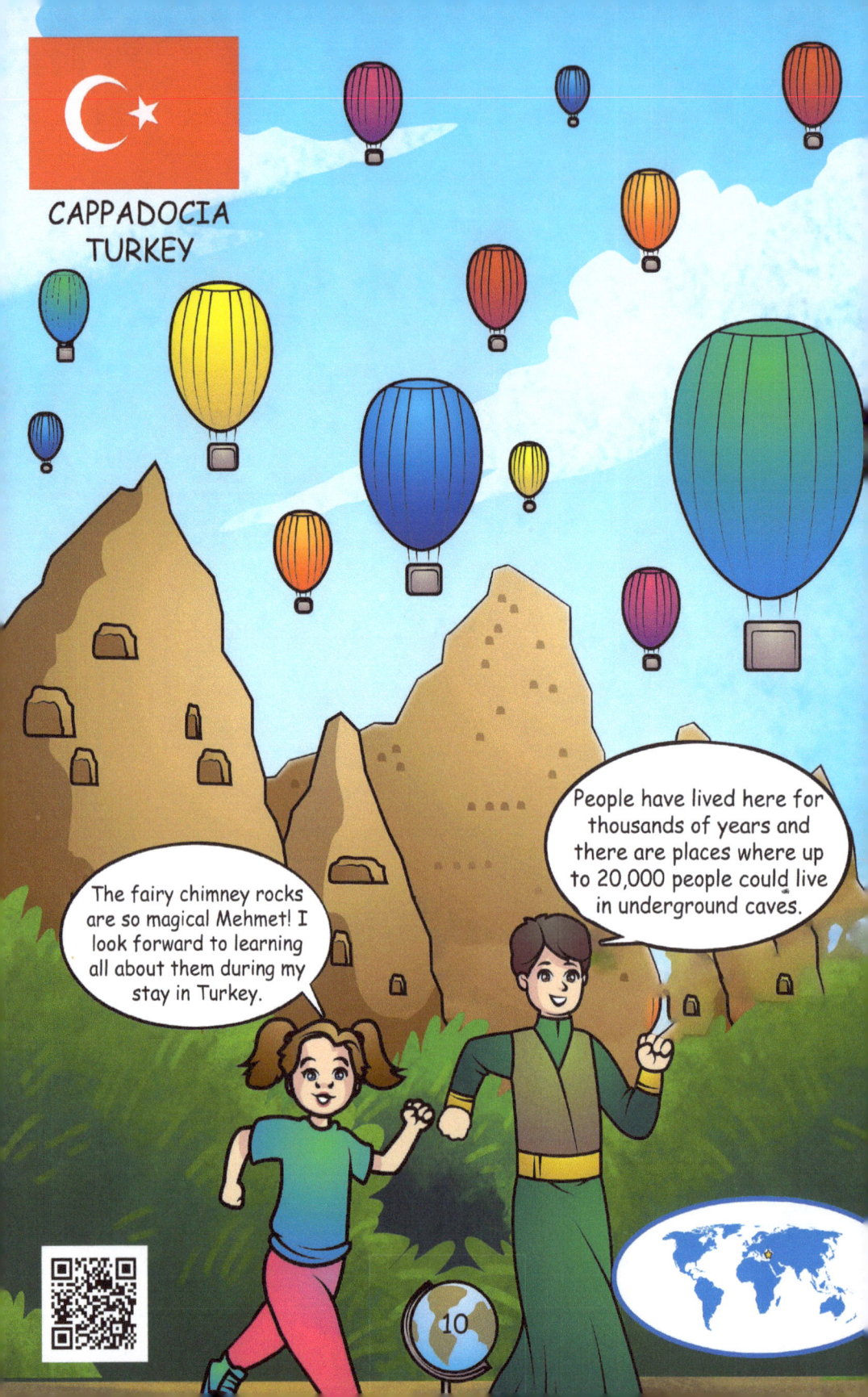

"The fairy chimney rocks are so magical Mehmet! I look forward to learning all about them during my stay in Turkey."

"People have lived here for thousands of years and there are places where up to 20,000 people could live in underground caves."

GUDVANGEN
NORWAY

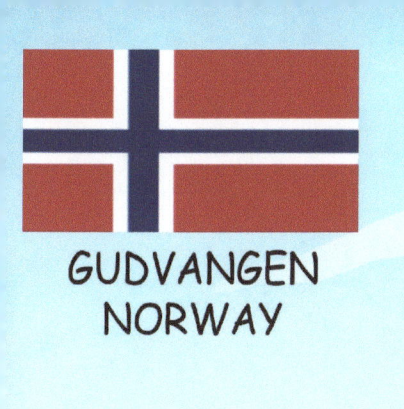

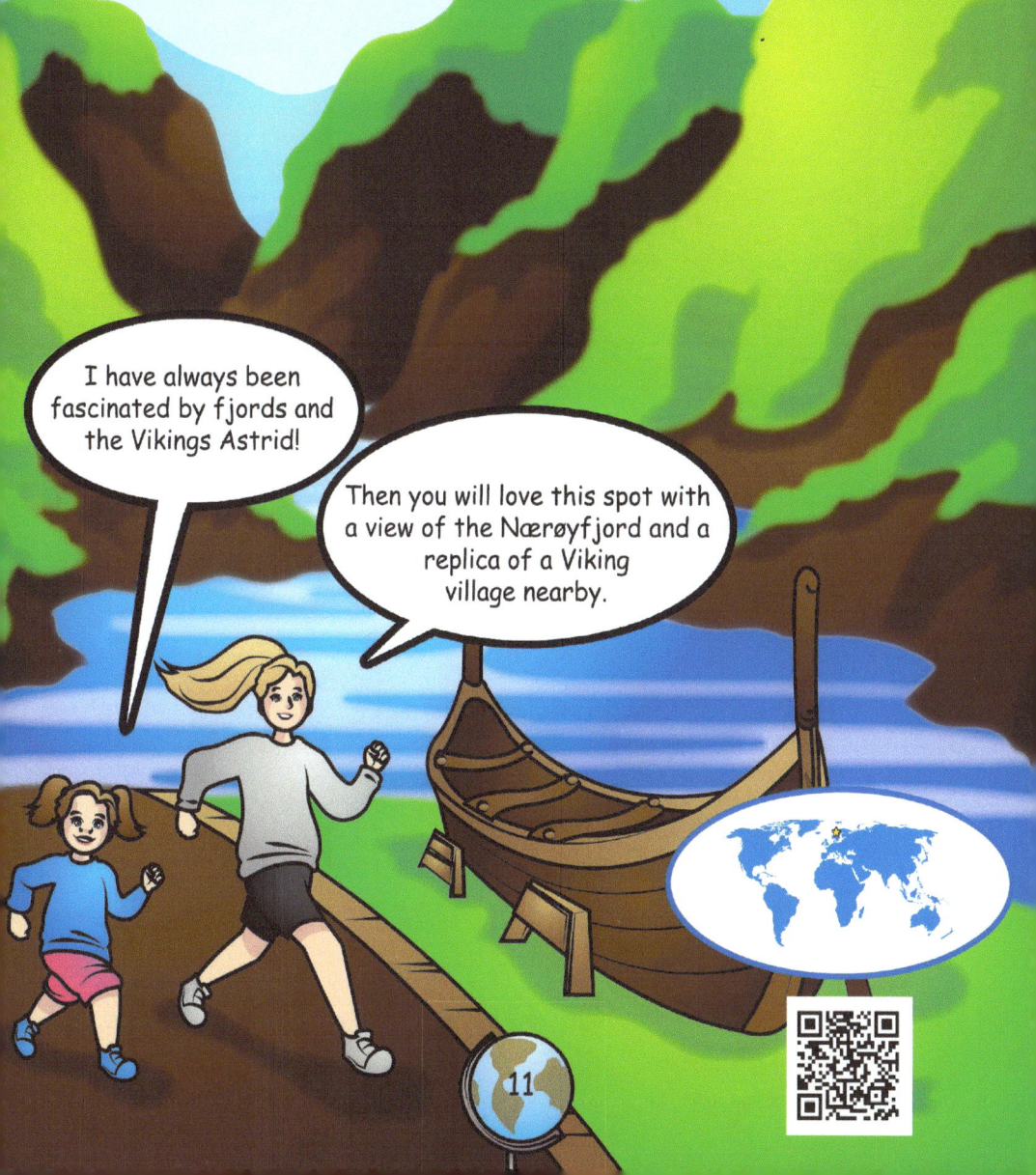

I have always been fascinated by fjords and the Vikings Astrid!

Then you will love this spot with a view of the Nærøyfjord and a replica of a Viking village nearby.

REYKJAVIK
ICELAND

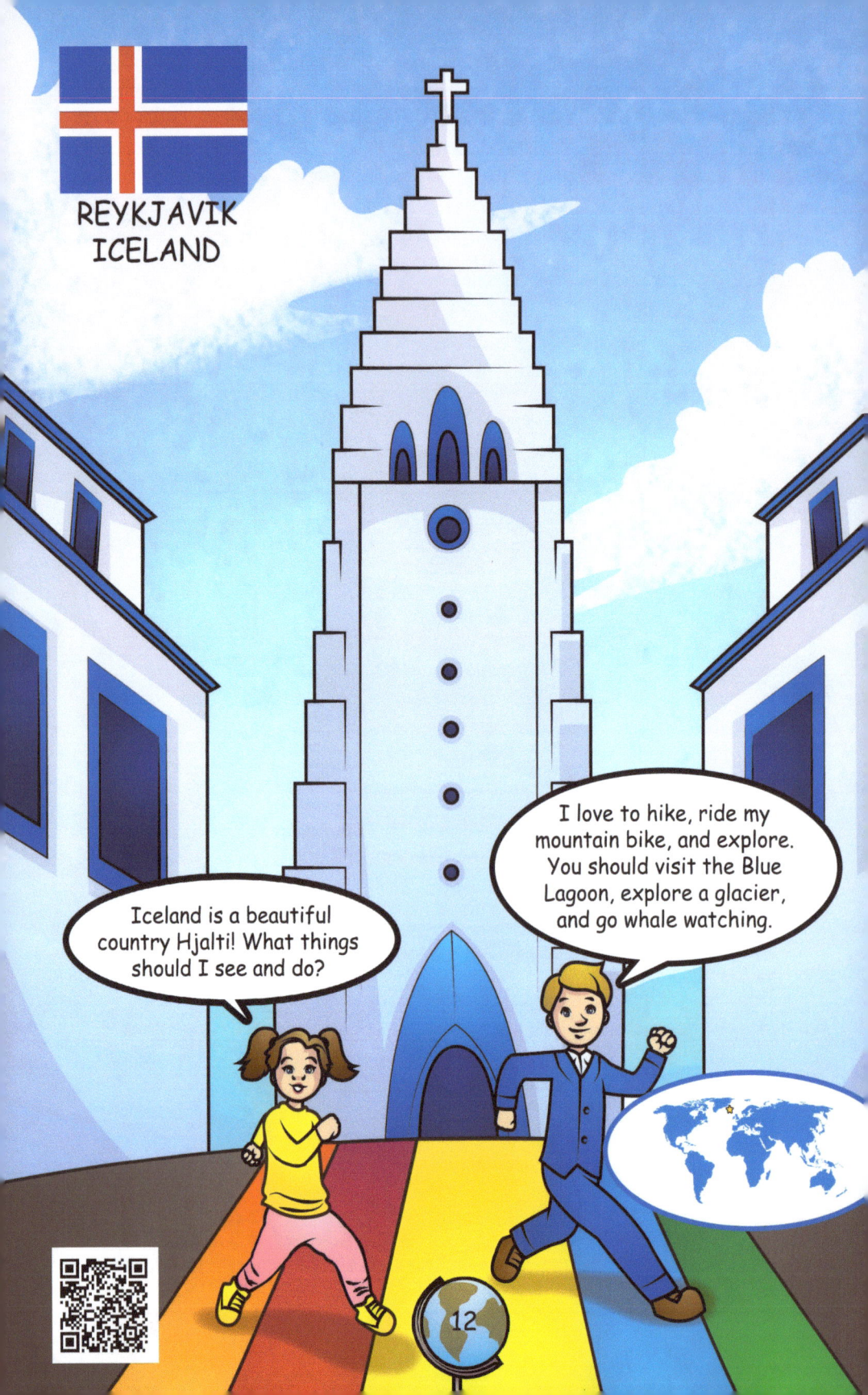

"Iceland is a beautiful country Hjalti! What things should I see and do?"

"I love to hike, ride my mountain bike, and explore. You should visit the Blue Lagoon, explore a glacier, and go whale watching."

12

ALCAZAR DE SEGOVIA
SPAIN

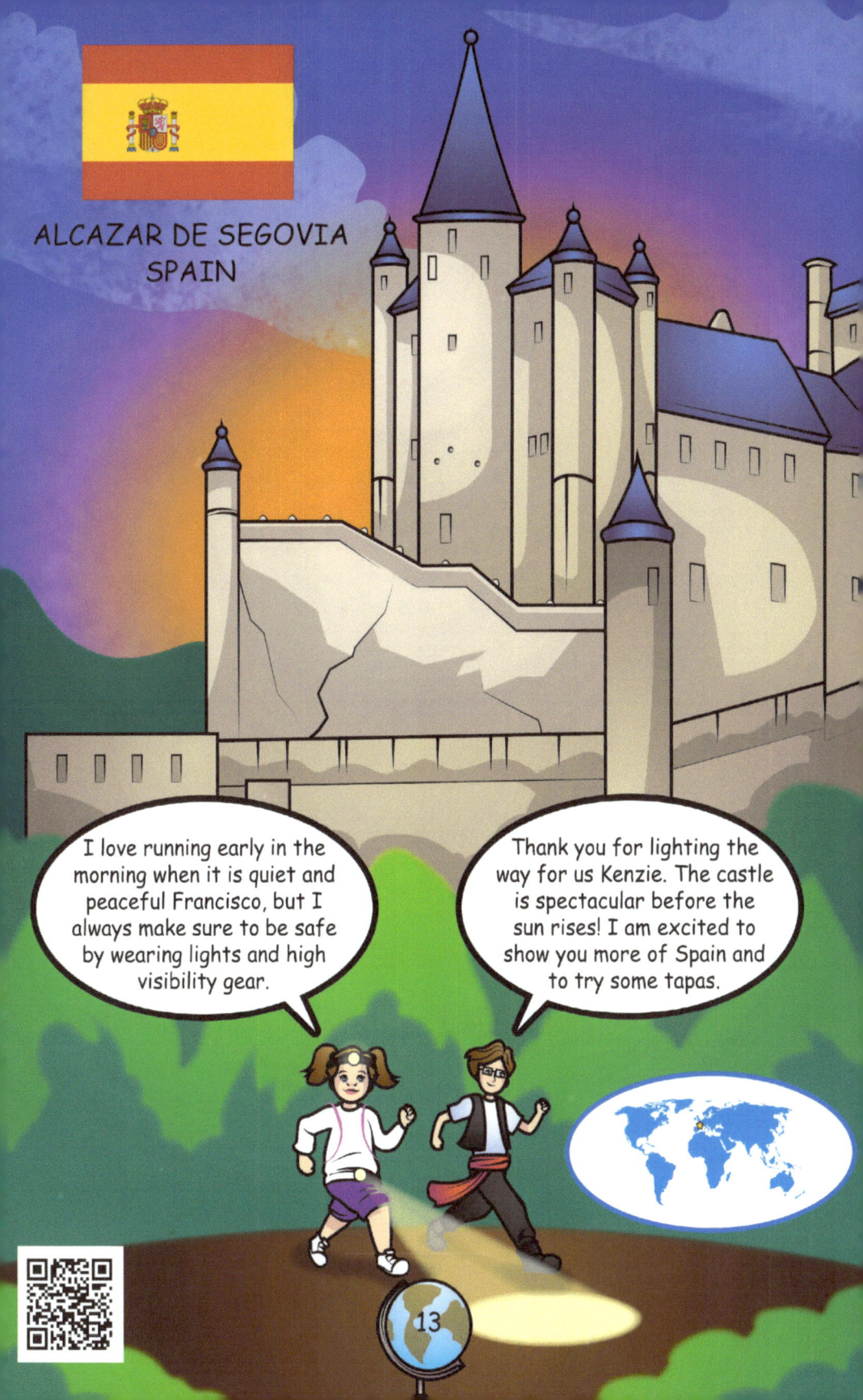

"I love running early in the morning when it is quiet and peaceful Francisco, but I always make sure to be safe by wearing lights and high visibility gear."

"Thank you for lighting the way for us Kenzie. The castle is spectacular before the sun rises! I am excited to show you more of Spain and to try some tapas."

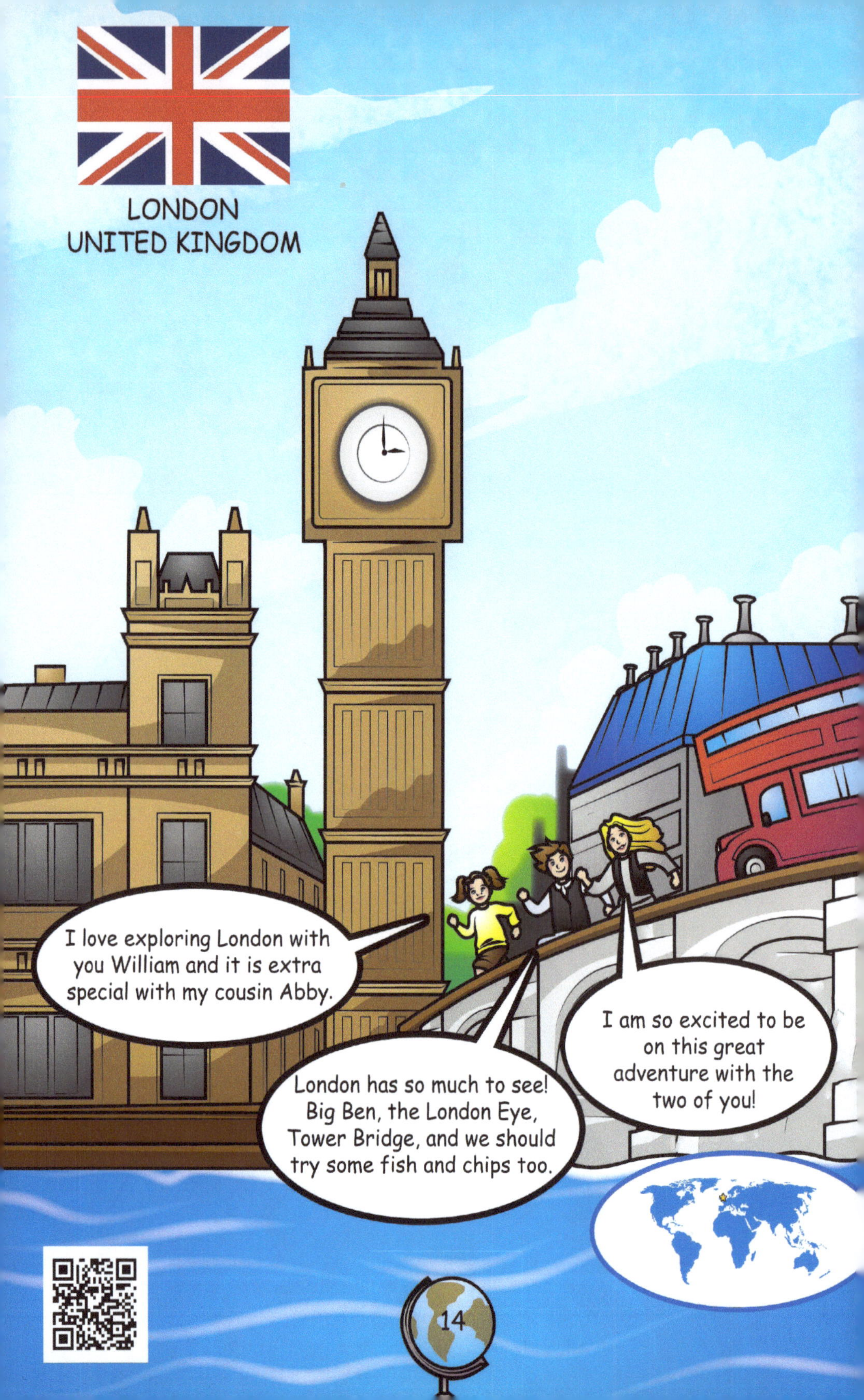
LONDON
UNITED KINGDOM
I love exploring London with you William and it is extra special with my cousin Abby.
London has so much to see! Big Ben, the London Eye, Tower Bridge, and we should try some fish and chips too.
I am so excited to be on this great adventure with the two of you!

PARIS
FRANCE

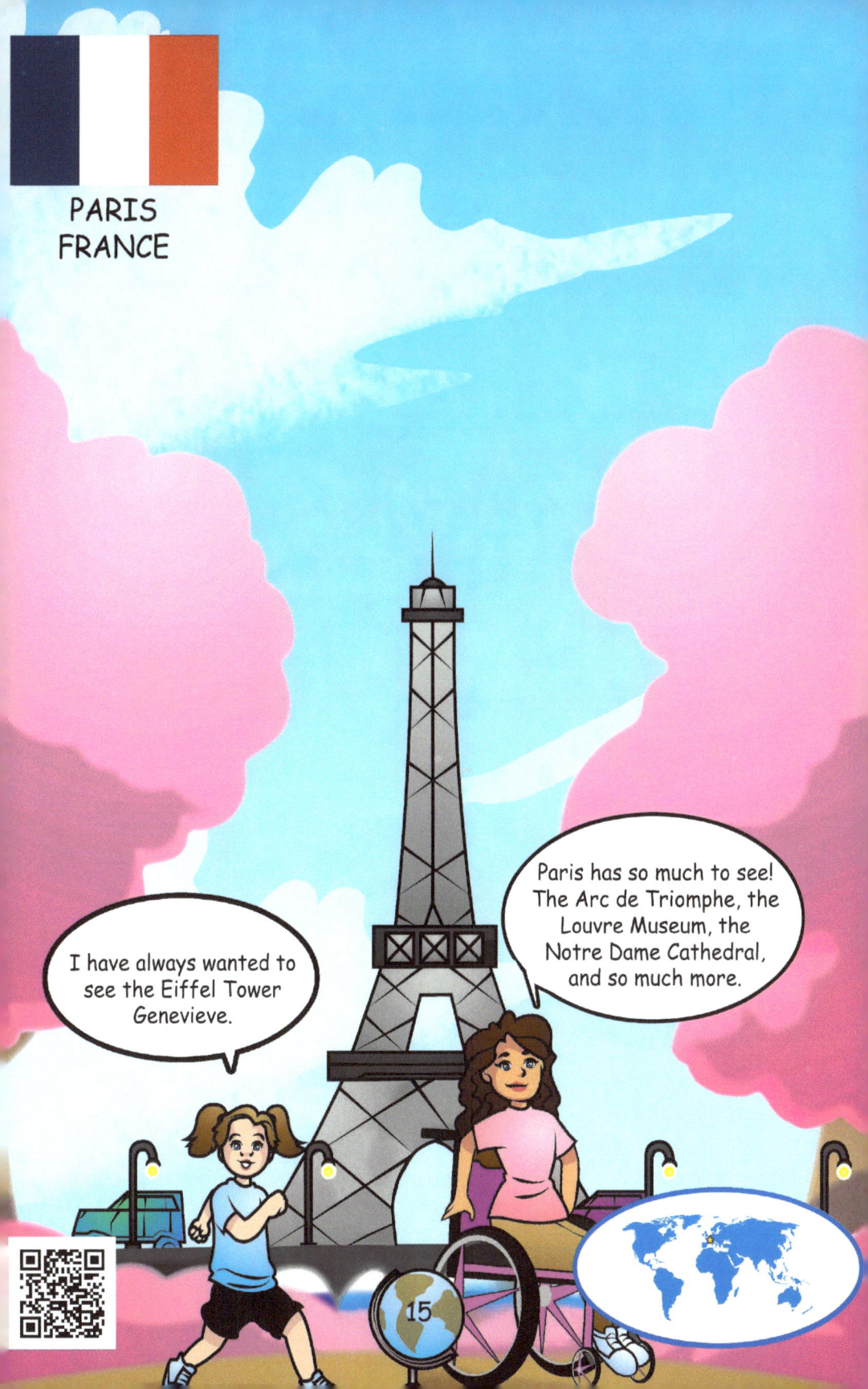

I have always wanted to see the Eiffel Tower Genevieve.

Paris has so much to see! The Arc de Triomphe, the Louvre Museum, the Notre Dame Cathedral, and so much more.

15

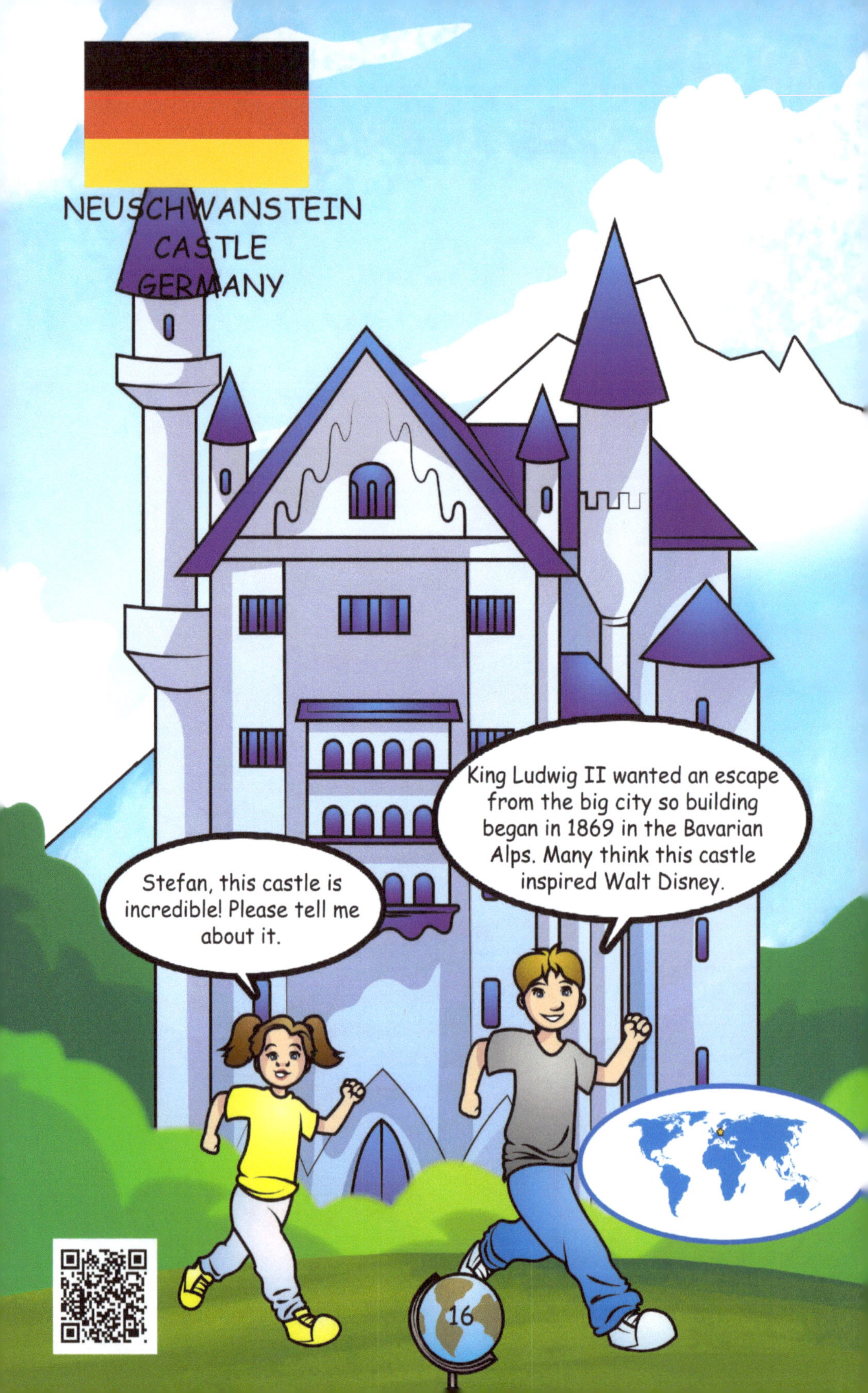
NEUSCHWANSTEIN
CASTLE
GERMANY
Stefan, this castle is incredible! Please tell me about it.
King Ludwig II wanted an escape from the big city so building began in 1869 in the Bavarian Alps. Many think this castle inspired Walt Disney.

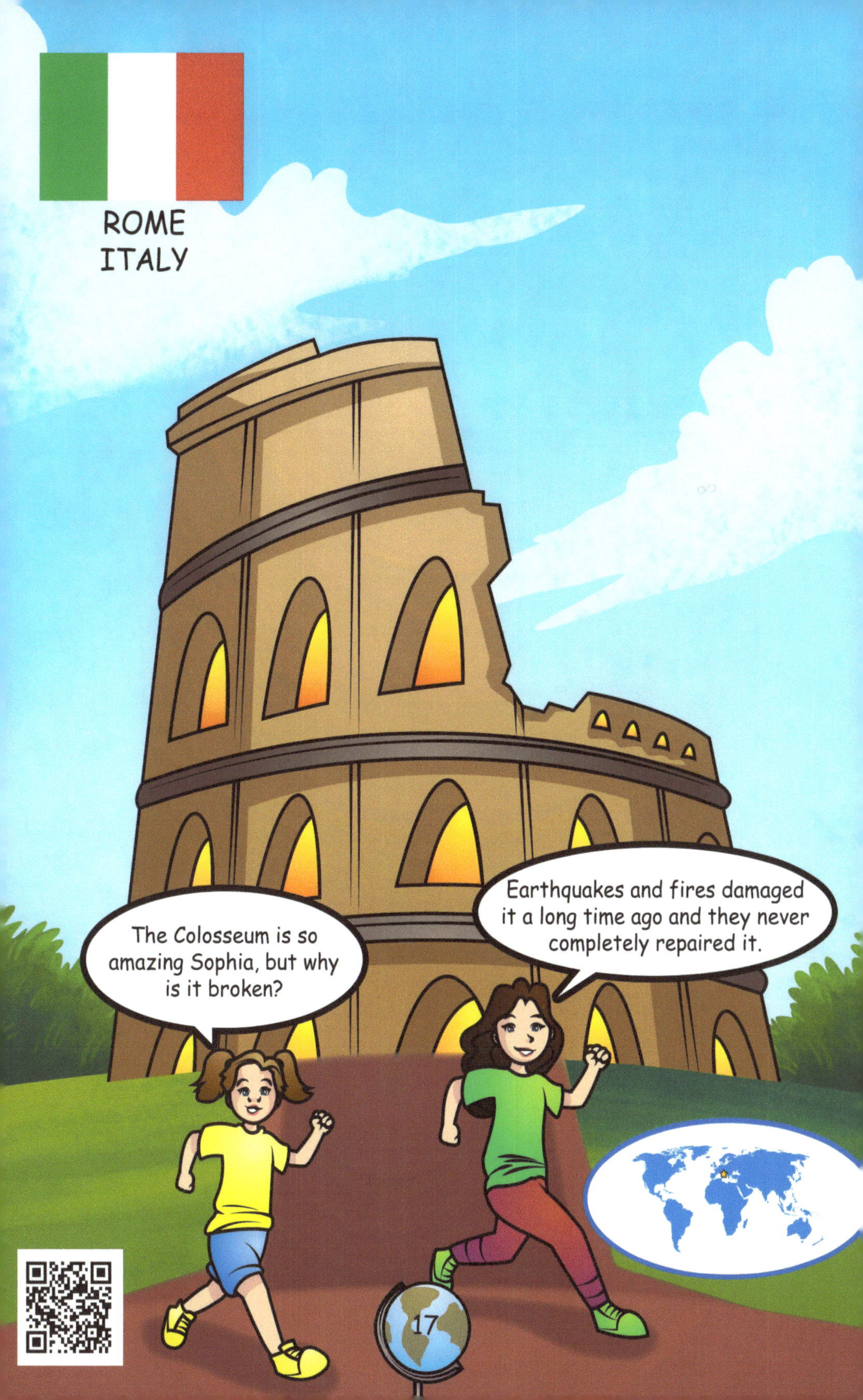
ROME
ITALY
The Colosseum is so amazing Sophia, but why is it broken?
Earthquakes and fires damaged it a long time ago and they never completely repaired it.

ATHENS GREECE

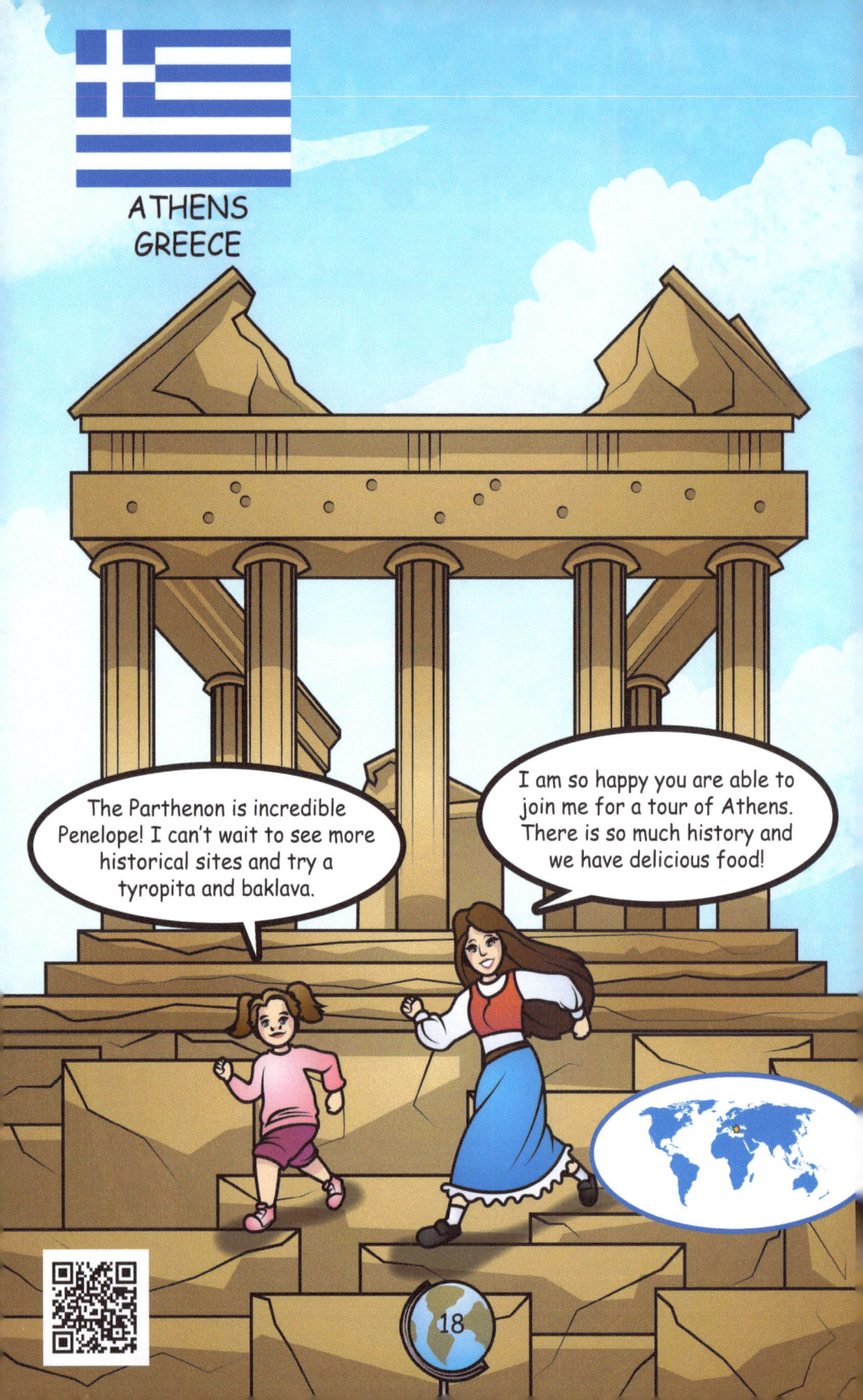

The Parthenon is incredible Penelope! I can't wait to see more historical sites and try a tyropita and baklava.

I am so happy you are able to join me for a tour of Athens. There is so much history and we have delicious food!

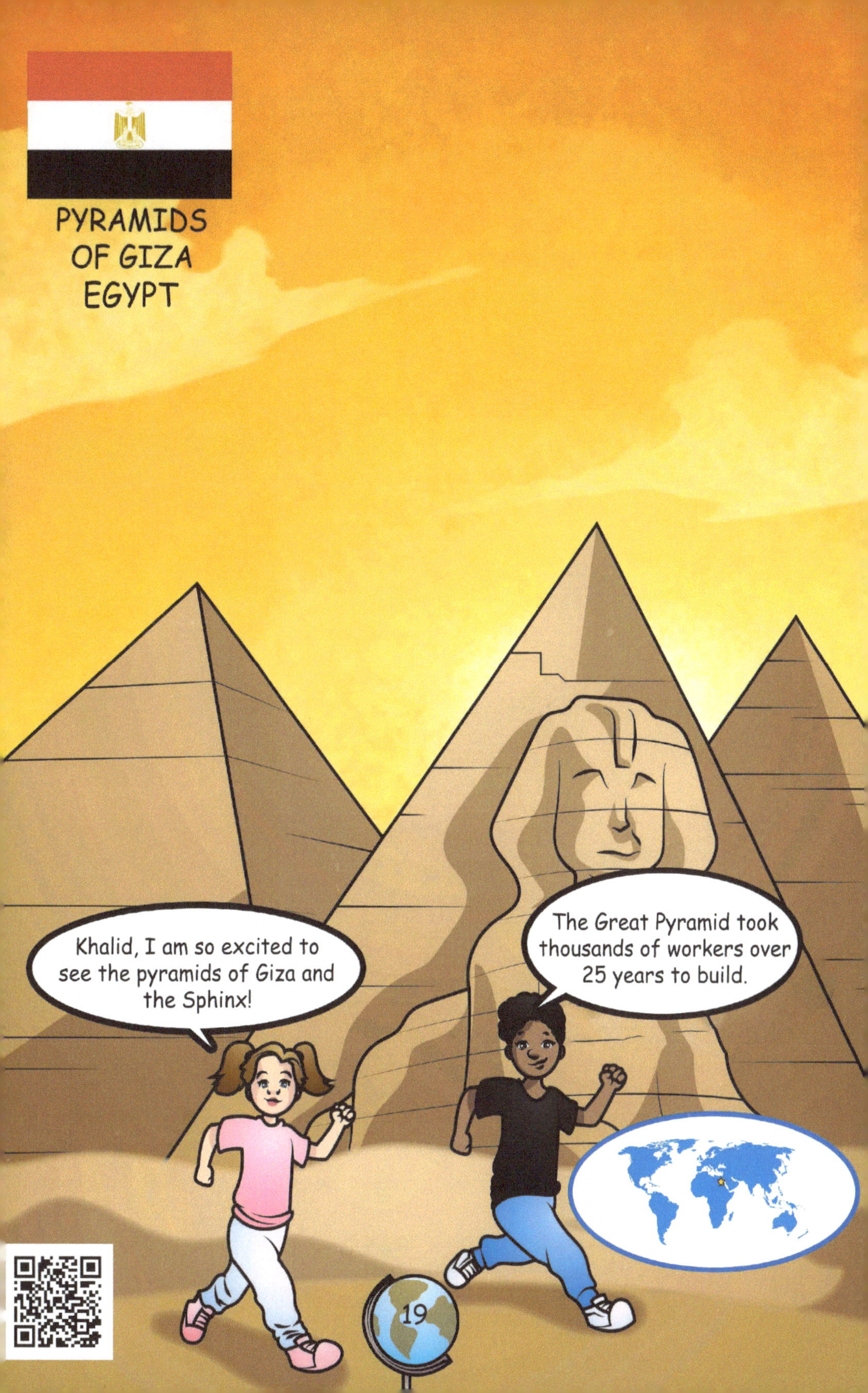
PYRAMIDS
OF GIZA
EGYPT
Khalid, I am so excited to see the pyramids of Giza and the Sphinx!
The Great Pyramid took thousands of workers over 25 years to build.
19

AMBOSELI
KENYA

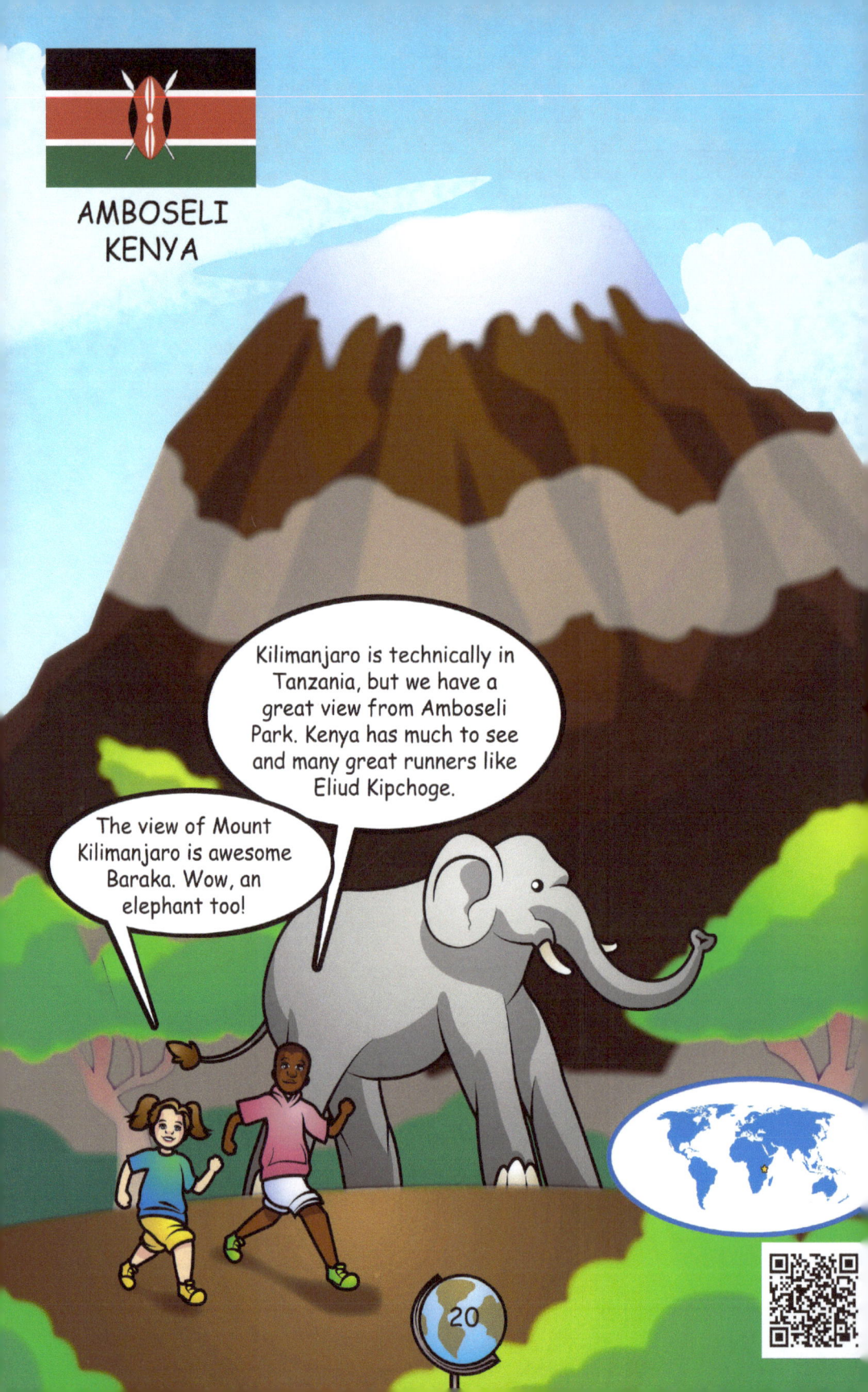

"Kilimanjaro is technically in Tanzania, but we have a great view from Amboseli Park. Kenya has much to see and many great runners like Eliud Kipchoge."

"The view of Mount Kilimanjaro is awesome Baraka. Wow, an elephant too!"

20

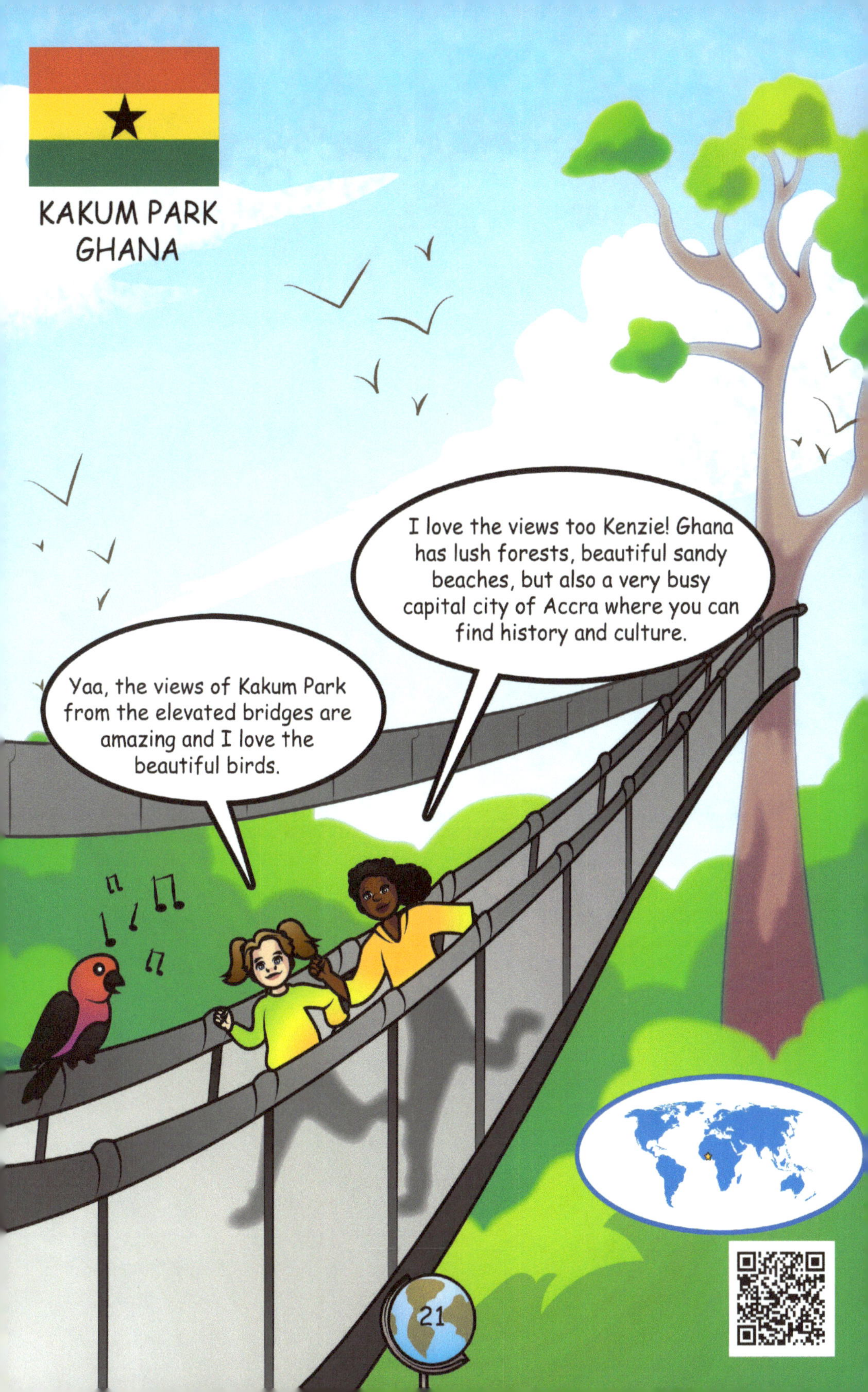
KAKUM PARK
GHANA
Yaa, the views of Kakum Park from the elevated bridges are amazing and I love the beautiful birds.
I love the views too Kenzie! Ghana has lush forests, beautiful sandy beaches, but also a very busy capital city of Accra where you can find history and culture.

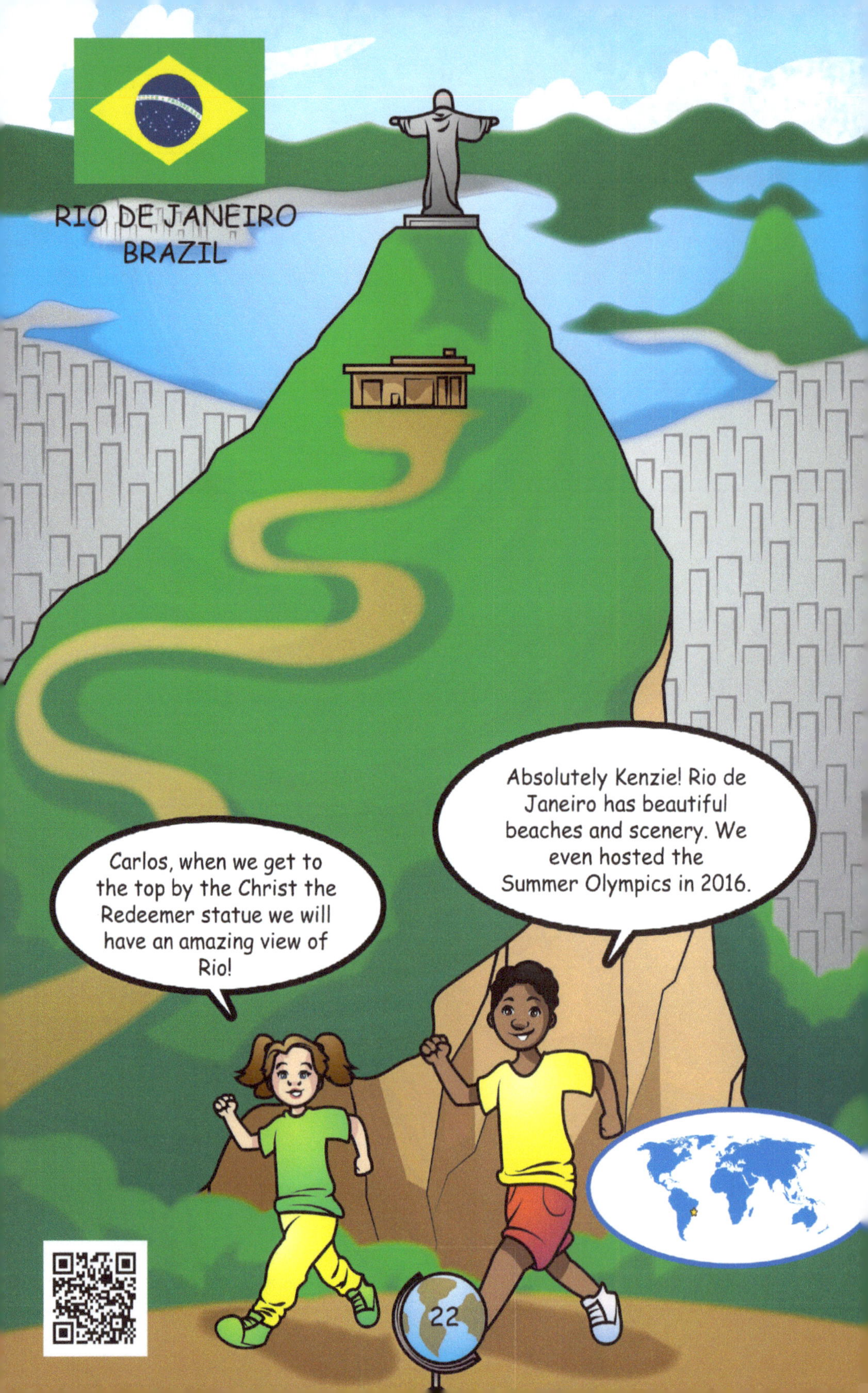
RIO DE JANEIRO
BRAZIL
Carlos, when we get to the top by the Christ the Redeemer statue we will have an amazing view of Rio!
Absolutely Kenzie! Rio de Janeiro has beautiful beaches and scenery. We even hosted the Summer Olympics in 2016.
22

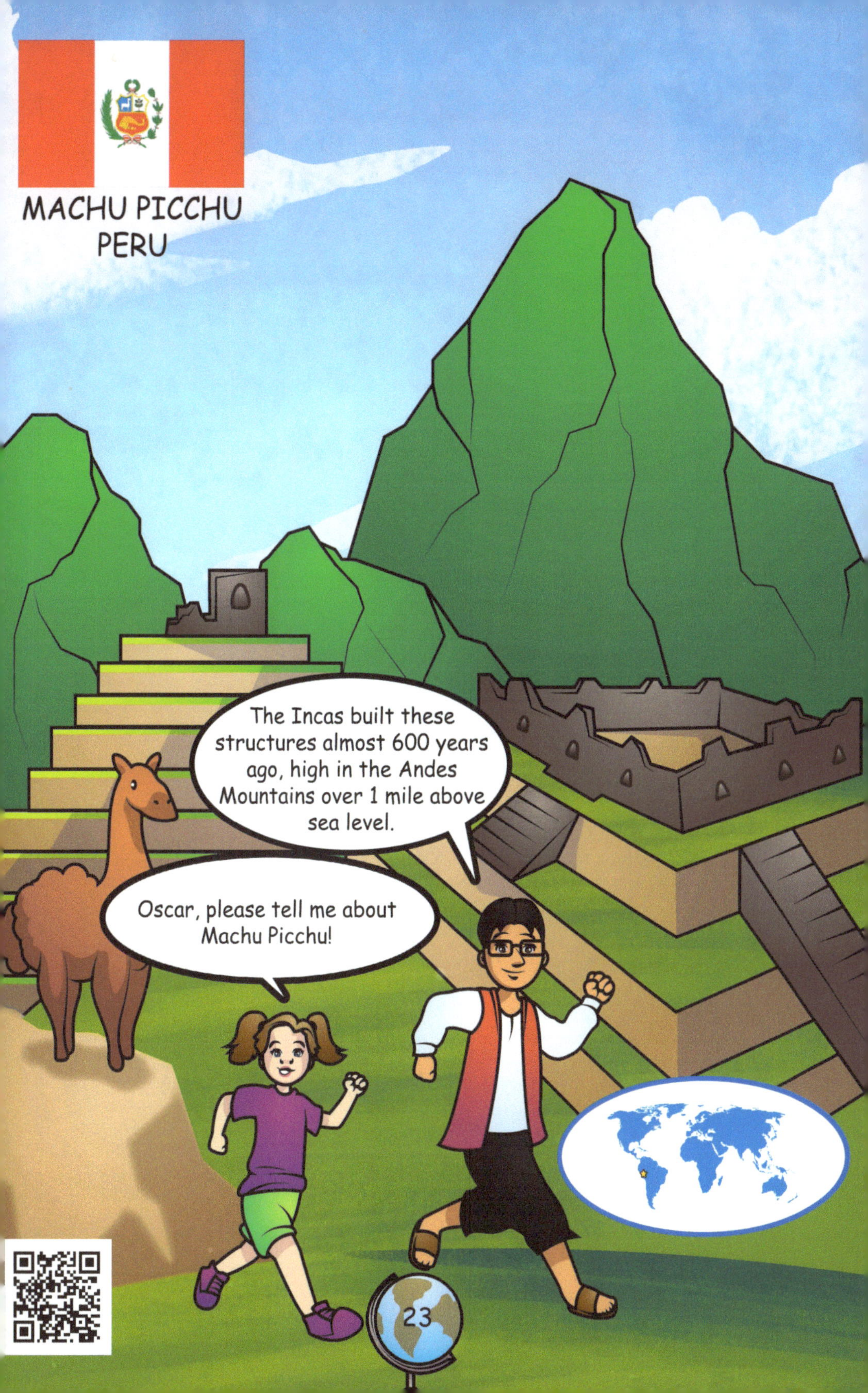
MACHU PICCHU
PERU
Oscar, please tell me about Machu Picchu!
The Incas built these structures almost 600 years ago, high in the Andes Mountains over 1 mile above sea level.

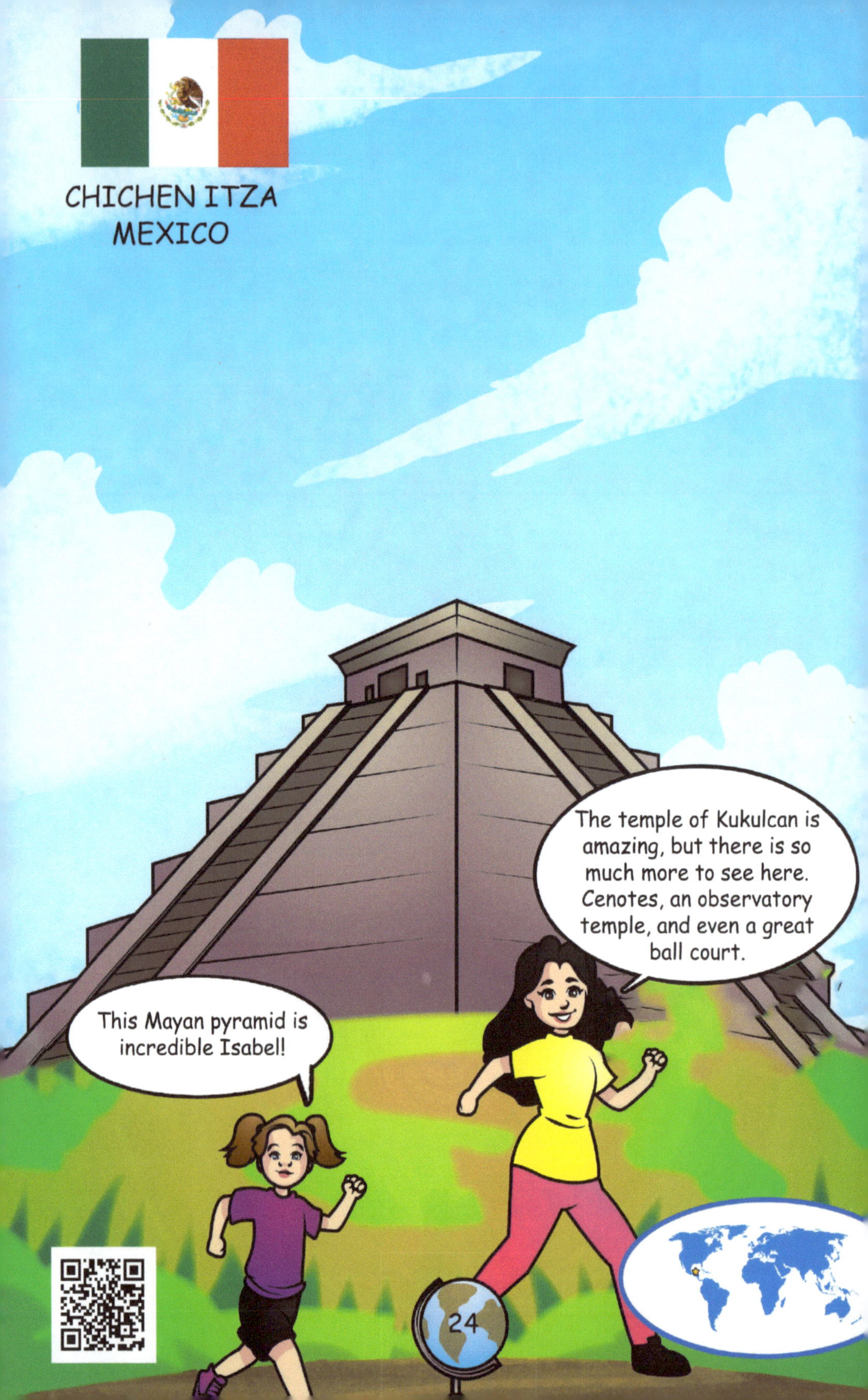
CHICHEN ITZA
MEXICO
The temple of Kukulcan is amazing, but there is so much more to see here. Cenotes, an observatory temple, and even a great ball court.
This Mayan pyramid is incredible Isabel!

WALT DISNEY
WORLD
USA

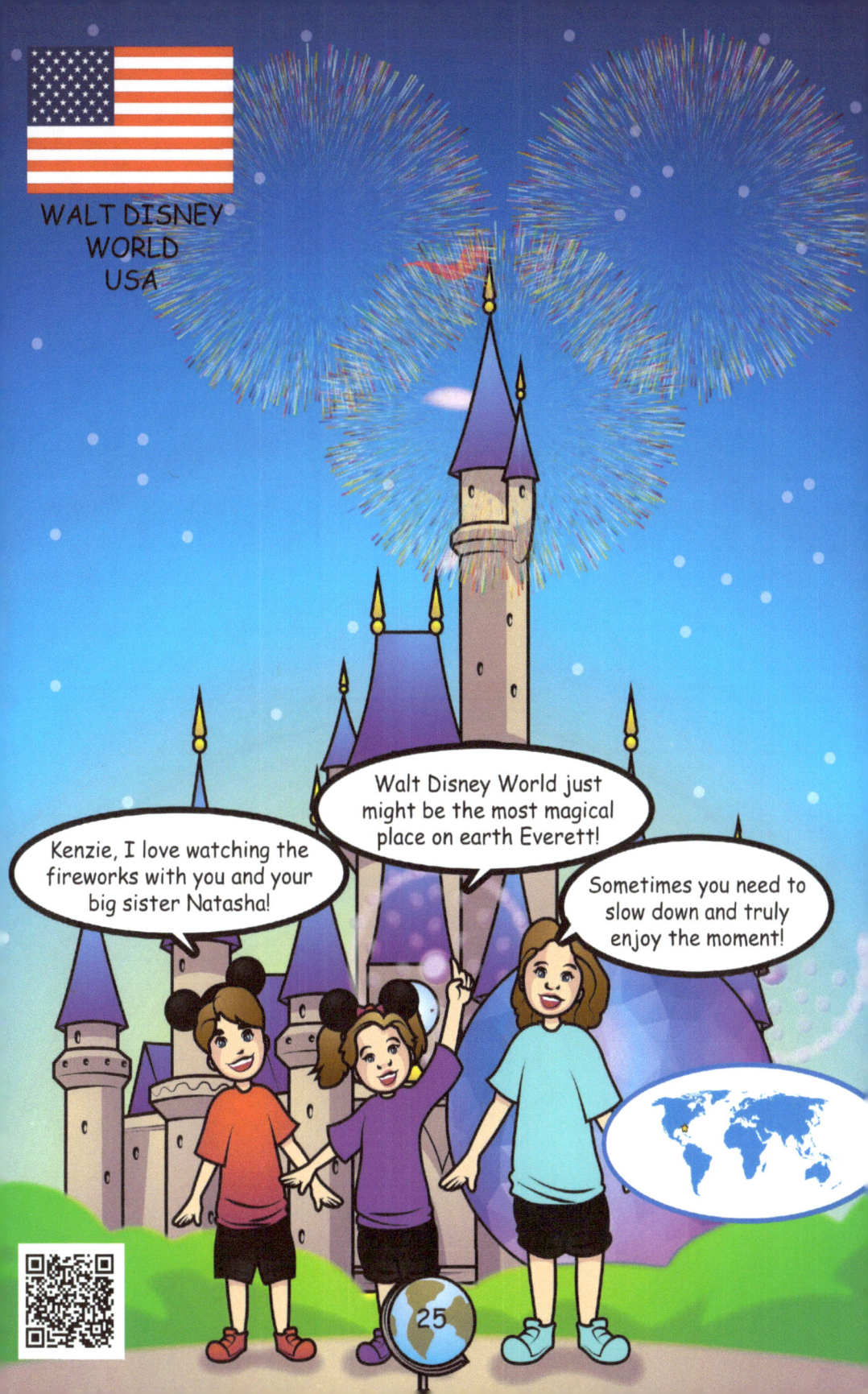

Kenzie, I love watching the fireworks with you and your big sister Natasha!

Walt Disney World just might be the most magical place on earth Everett!

Sometimes you need to slow down and truly enjoy the moment!

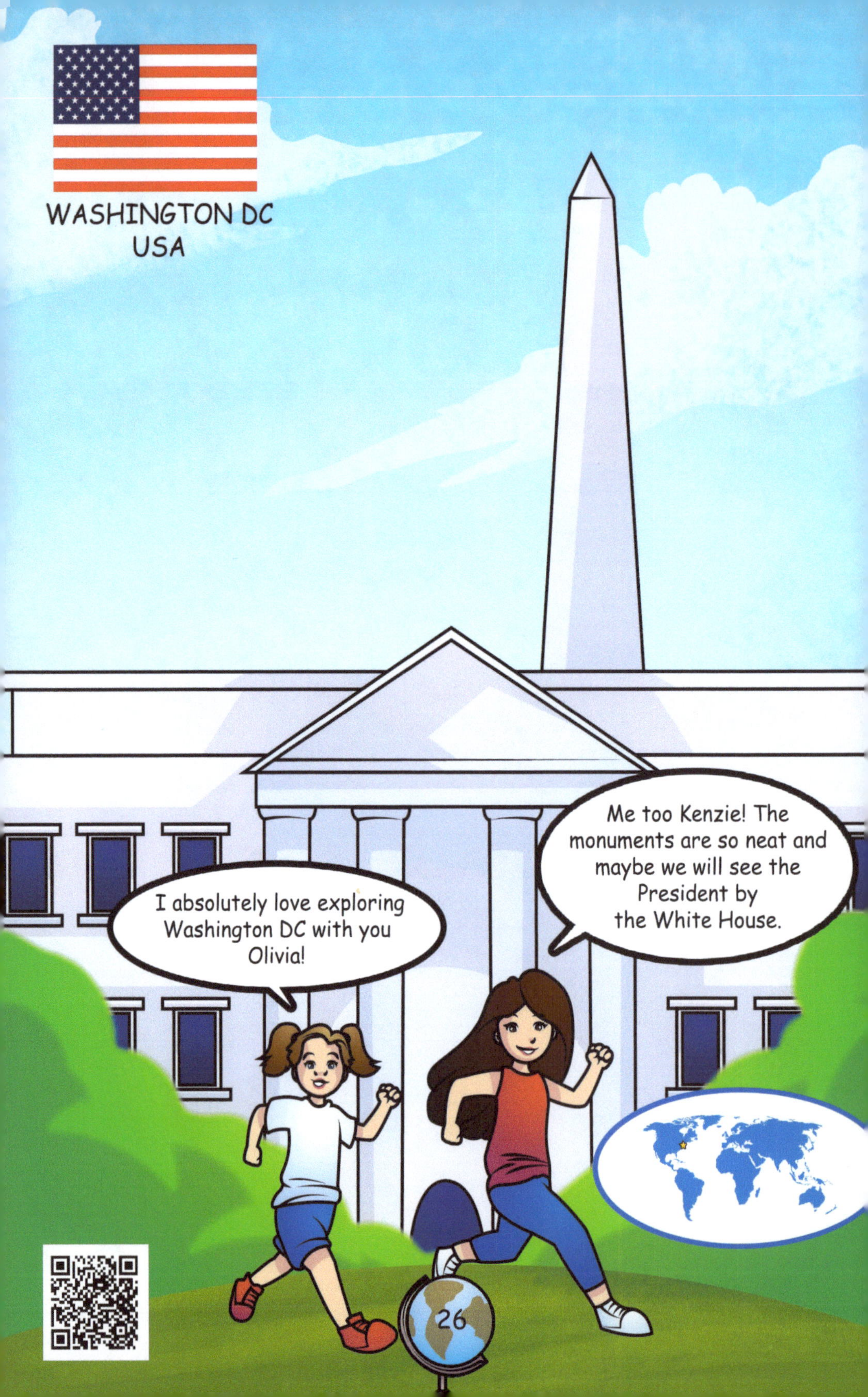
WASHINGTON DC
USA
I absolutely love exploring Washington DC with you Olivia!
Me too Kenzie! The monuments are so neat and maybe we will see the President by the White House.
26

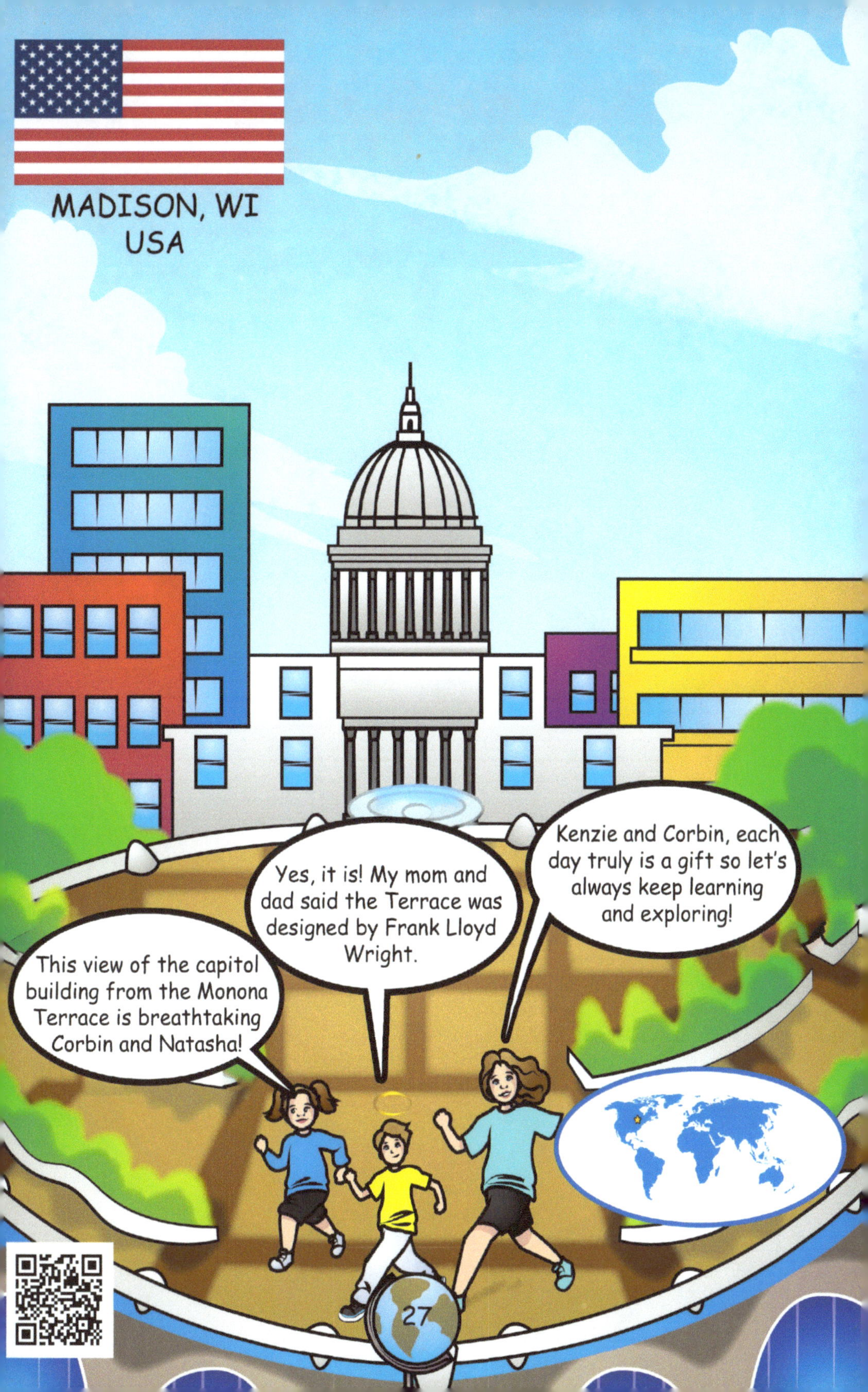
MADISON, WI
USA
This view of the capitol building from the Monona Terrace is breathtaking Corbin and Natasha!
Yes, it is! My mom and dad said the Terrace was designed by Frank Lloyd Wright.
Kenzie and Corbin, each day truly is a gift so let's always keep learning and exploring!

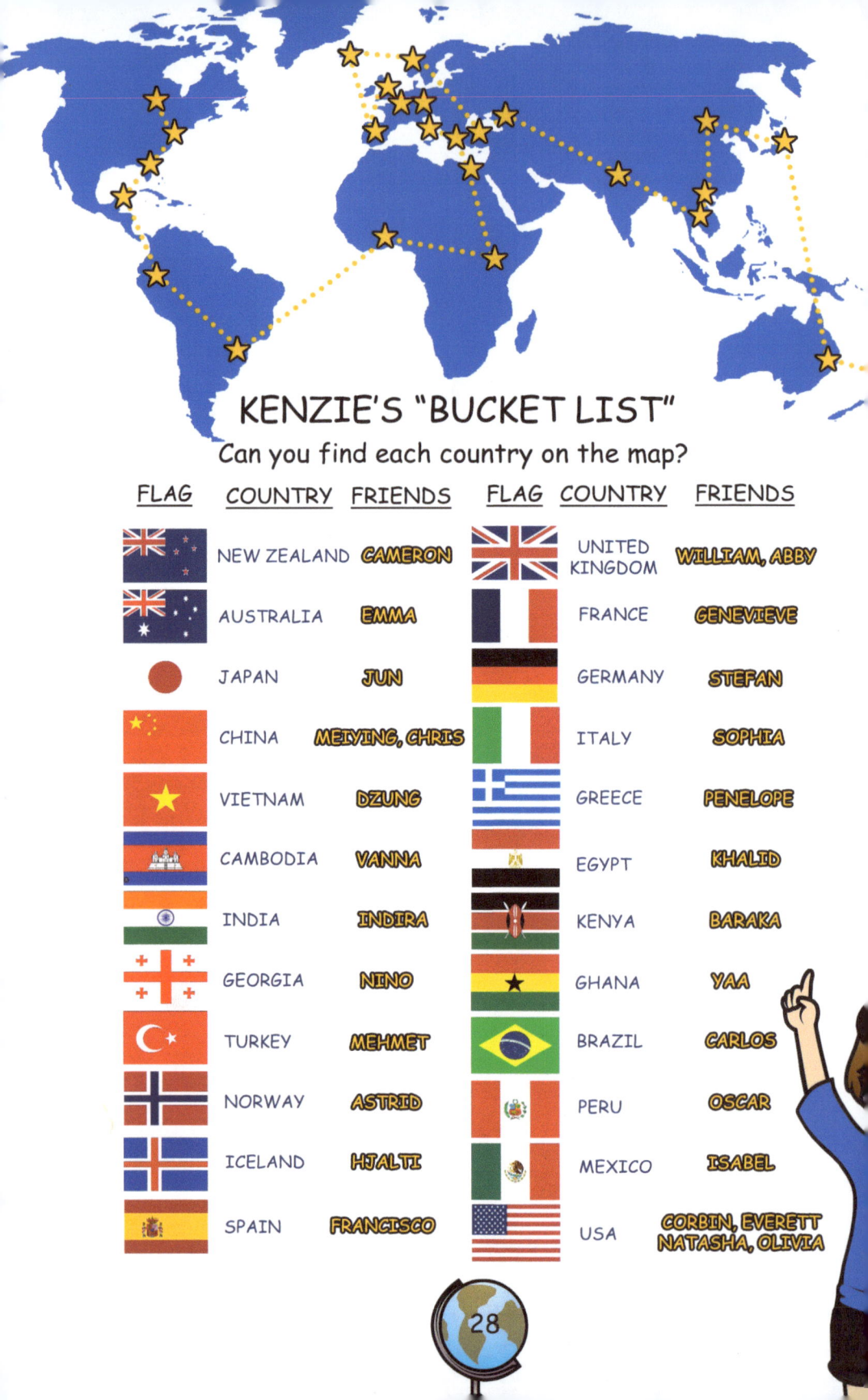

KENZIE'S "BUCKET LIST"
Can you find each country on the map?

FLAG	COUNTRY	FRIENDS	FLAG	COUNTRY	FRIENDS
	NEW ZEALAND	CAMERON		UNITED KINGDOM	WILLIAM, ABBY
	AUSTRALIA	EMMA		FRANCE	GENEVIEVE
	JAPAN	JUN		GERMANY	STEFAN
	CHINA	MEIYING, CHRIS		ITALY	SOPHIA
	VIETNAM	DZUNG		GREECE	PENELOPE
	CAMBODIA	VANNA		EGYPT	KHALID
	INDIA	INDIRA		KENYA	BARAKA
	GEORGIA	NINO		GHANA	YAA
	TURKEY	MEHMET		BRAZIL	CARLOS
	NORWAY	ASTRID		PERU	OSCAR
	ICELAND	HJALTI		MEXICO	ISABEL
	SPAIN	FRANCISCO		USA	CORBIN, EVERETT, NATASHA, OLIVIA

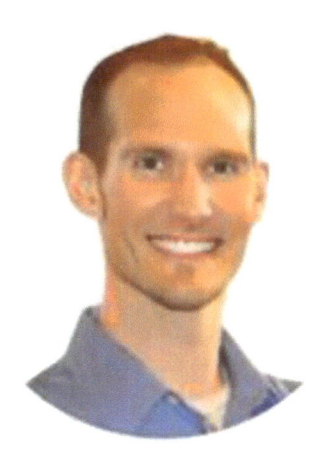

ABOUT THE AUTHOR

Brian Cleven is a father, husband, Race Director, 13-time IRONMAN Triathlon Finisher and counting, and has run at least 1 continuous mile each day since July 2nd, 2010. (Over 5,170 days in a row) From the small town of Peshtigo, Wisconsin he earned his bachelor's and master's degrees at the University of Wisconsin-La Crosse. As an ACSM Certified Clinical Exercise Physiologist and Licensed Athletic Trainer he leads a Cardiopulmonary Rehabilitation program and performs Cardiac Stress Testing at the Emplify Health Marinette Clinic and was named the 2024 Certified Professional of the Year by the American College of Sports Medicine. In his free time, you will find him enjoying his family, traveling, writing, training for his next race, or partnering with other community members to provide opportunities for people to become the healthiest versions of themselves!

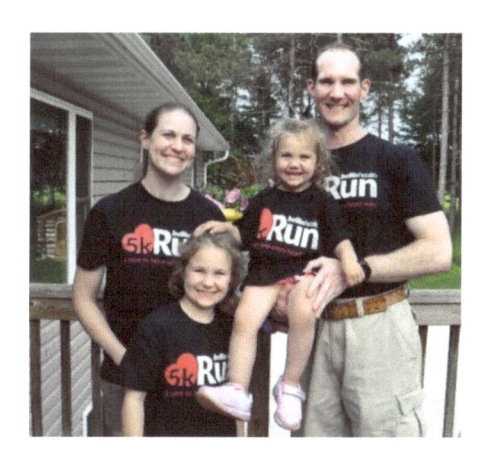

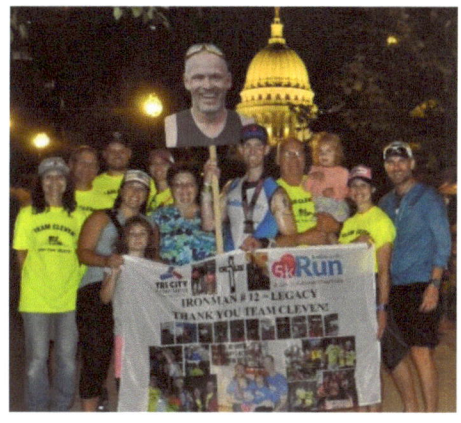

COMING SOON...

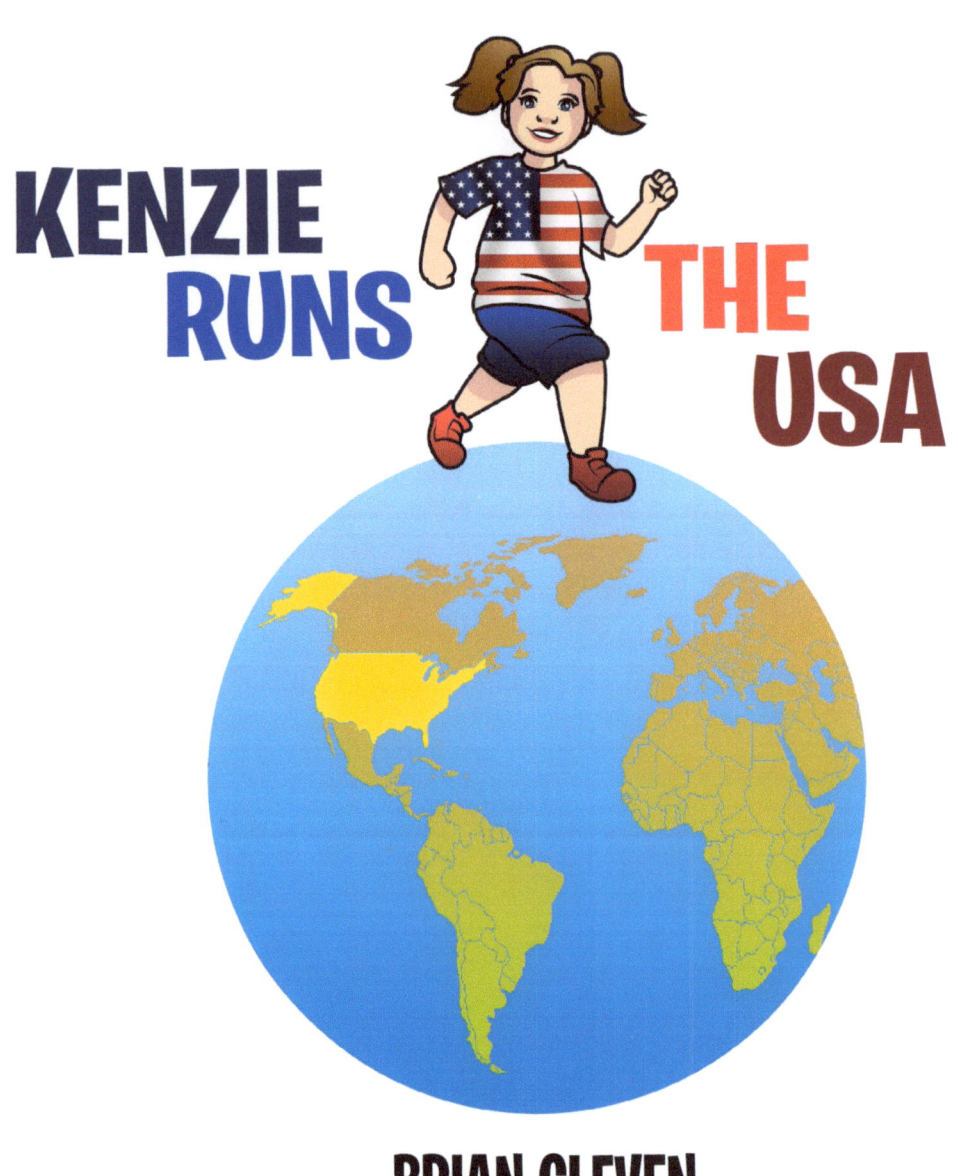

KENZIE RUNS THE USA

BRIAN CLEVEN

Printed in the USA
CPSIA information can be obtained
at www.ICGtesting.com
LVHW071321301124
797836LV00001B/8